Sadye L. Logan, DSW, ACSW
Edith M. Freeman, PhD, ACSW
Editors

Health Care in the Black Community
Empowerment, Knowledge, Skills, and Collectivism

Pre-publication
REVIEWS,
COMMENTARIES,
EVALUATIONS . . .

"**R**eaders in search of an authoritative source on the topic of African-American health care can now breathe a sigh of relief. *Health Care in the Black Community: Empowerment, Knowledge, Skills, and Collectivism* is a valuable resource for academicians, students, social service practitioners, clinicians, medical professionals, or anyone interested in the health and well-being of the African-American community. Readers are reminded of the health care issues of concern to this community, but more important, they are given a refreshing, alternative worldview from which to map a course of intervention. This worldview is holistic, emphasizing physical and mental health, elderly and adolescent issues, and clinical and macro interventions, and gives voice to spiritual as well as scientific notions. Many of the chapters provide practical diagrams that elucidate comprehensive models of intervention. In addition, case illustrations provide rich examples of health care concerns and illuminate the proper application of theoretical frameworks. This book is a must read for all."

Ramona Denby, PhD
Assistant Professor,
University of Nevada
School of Social Work,
Las Vegas

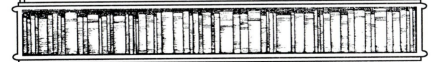

"**T**his is a must-read book for those who take seriously the practical and practice sides of health care in African-American communities. The scholarship represented in the content realistically develops from strength and empowerment modalities. Additionally, through the use of success stories of lives with difficult circumstances, the writers effectively negate media-hyped negative stereotypes of this population.

Readers will benefit in several ways. They will be (a) oriented to authentic ways of thinking about African-American health care, (b) better prepared to develop realistic intervention strategies, and (c) more efficiently equipped to implement such strategies.

The book is an integrative whole with excellent opening and concluding paragraphs by the editors. The chapters each contain excellent models/paradigms that are transferable to non-health related areas of practice. Educators, practitioners, and administrators will find various aspects of the book useful."

Brenda K. J. Crawley, PhD
Associate Professor,
Loyola University Chicago
School of Social Work

"**A**s a social work educator, I am coming across more students who now seek alternative approaches to problem solving; they are interested in working within communities and with community-based agents for social change. They seek creative approaches to tackling problems that confront not just a few but many—they need the orientation to problem analysis and the proactive responsive strategies put forth in *Health Care in the Black Community: Empowerment, Knowledge, Skills, and Collectivism* by Drs. Sadye L. Logan and Edith M. Freeman. This text fills the gap in the literature by providing pragmatic approaches to tackling the health care crisis in the black community. The strategies, focusing on collectivism and family-centered approaches to problem definition and problem solving, are transferable to other need areas as well.

In addition to the emphasis on family-focused strategies for change that are community generated, I like the focus on early intervention approaches and a commitment to prevention that are carried throughout the book, whether discussing the Black Church and mental health or early parenthood among young, black fathers. Partnerships is another focal characteristic of successful interventions aimed at improving the health care status—the survival status—of the African-American community."

Carla M. Curtis, PhD
Associate Professor,
The Ohio State University
College of Social Work

More pre-publication
REVIEWS, COMMENTARIES, EVALUATIONS . . .

"**F**or more than a decade, Logan and Freeman's collaborations have yielded rich descriptions of how social work practice can effectively serve African-American communities. Their newest volume, *Health Care in the Black Community*, is no exception. Logan and Freeman present a model based upon Barbara Solomon's fundamental conceptualization of empowerment. Recognizing that critical consciousness and confidence are realized through analysis and new skill development, they demonstrate how African-American individuals, families, groups, and communities can build health-promoting connections. Scholars from nursing, psychology, medicine, and social work provide excellent illustrations of how the model addresses several risk factors of vital importance within African-American communities, including the growing aging population, family violence, HIV/ AIDS, early parenthood, and limited compliance with medication regimes.

Chapters devoted to infertility, spirituality, and contemporary churches in African-American communities are of particular note because of the limited literature combining theory, research, and practice in these areas.

Another major contribution of this book is its attention to often used and seldom operationalized conceptual frameworks and concepts in social work practice. Chapters addressing ethnoconscious approaches to reality therapy, individual and family strengths enhancement, cognitive-behavioral intervention, stress and coping, and community-building increase our understanding of functional social work roles within African-American communities. This integrative text will be an invaluable tool for social work faculty, students, and practitioners."

Edith A. Lewis, MSW, PhD
*Associate Professor of Social Work,
University of Michigan*

The Haworth Press, Inc.

Health Care in the Black Community
Empowerment, Knowledge, Skills, and Collectivism

HAWORTH SOCIAL WORK IN HEALTH CARE
Gary Rosenberg and Andrew Weissman
Editors

A Guide to Creative Group Programming in the Psychiatric Day Hospital by Lois E. Passi

Social Work in Geriatric Home Health Care: The Blending of Traditional Practice with Cooperative Strategies by Lucille Rosengarten

Health Care in the Black Community: Empowerment, Knowledge, Skills, and Collectivism edited by Sadye L. Logan and Edith M. Freeman

Health Care
in the Black Community
Empowerment, Knowledge, Skills, and Collectivism

Sadye L. Logan, DSW, ACSW
Edith M. Freeman, PhD, ACSW
Editors

The Haworth Press®
New York • London • Oxford

The Haworth Press, Inc., 10 Alice Street, Binghamton, NY 13904-1580

DISCLAIMER
The case studies and vignettes presented in this book are based on actual clinical cases. However, all names, genders, and ages have been changed to protect the privacy of those individuals.

Cover design by Monica L. Seifert.

Library of Congress Cataloging-in-Publication Data

Health care in the Black community : empowerment, knowledge, skills, and collectivism / Sadye L. Logan, Edith M. Freeman, editors.
    p. cm.
  Includes bibliographical references and index.
  ISBN 0-7890-0456-9 (hard : alk. paper) — ISBN 0-7890-0457-7 (soft : alk. paper)
    1. Afro-Americans—Health and hygiene. 2. Afro-Americans—Medical care. 3. Health services accessibility—United States. I. Logan, Sadye Louise, date. II. Freeman, Edith M.

RA448.5.N4 H385 2000
362.1′089′96073—dc21
                                     00-038882

CONTENTS

PART IV: EPILOGUE

ABOUT THE EDITORS

Sadye L. Logan, DSW, MSW, formerly of the University of Kansas, Lawrence, Kansas, where she chaired the foundation practice sequence and co-chaired the Institute for the Study of Black Families, currently holds the I. De Quincy Newman Endowed Professorship in Social Justice at the University of South Carolina College of Social Work. She teaches practice method courses and courses on family treatment. Her research interests include social justice issues impacting families and children, culturally specific services for children and families of color, the psychospiritual dimensions of practice and education, addictive behaviors, and racial identity development. Dr. Logan has written and published extensively in these areas. She has also addressed them through consultation; workshops; local, national, and international presentations; and professional organizations. Dr. Logan earned her MSW degree from Hunter College and her DSW from Columbia University, both in New York City.

Edith M. Freeman, PhD, MSW, is a professor and director of the doctoral program at the University of Kansas School of Social Welfare, Lawrence, Kansas, where she teaches graduate practice courses in the doctoral and master's programs. She was a recipient of the first Chancellor's Award for Teaching Excellence in 1989. Her writing and research interests include issues related to children and families, substance abuse prevention and treatment, multiculturalism, community development, and empowerment. Dr. Freeman has written eight books, numerous articles, and several training manuals in these areas. She earned her MSW and a PhD in Human Development and Family Life from the University of Kansas. She also provides consultation and training in these and other areas to staff members of community organizations and social agencies.

CONTRIBUTORS

Freda Brashears is a PhD candidate and has been a practicing social worker for thirty years, with a private practice in Kansas City, Missouri, while continuing to serve as a volunteer consultant and service provider for the social services program at Second Baptist Church. She is completing the PhD program at the University of Kansas School of Social Welfare, Lawrence, Kansas, for which her dissertation topic is "The Use of Spirituality in Health Crisis and Death: Narratives from Elderly African Americans." Future goals include teaching social workers at the college level and continuing to further the profession through theory and program development.

Edna Comer is an assistant professor in the School of Social Work at the University of Connecticut, Storrs, Connecticut. She served as a research assistant in the Psychosocial Research Division of Duke-UNC Comprehensive Sickle Cell Center. One of her research interests includes the development of group treatment strategies for depression in individuals with sickle cell disease. Other areas of interest include establishing and evaluating family support programs, African-American families, and intervention research. She received her MSW from Western Michigan University, Kalamazoo, Michigan, and her PhD from the University of North Carolina at Chapel Hill.

M. Jenise Comer is an associate professor of Social Work at Central Missouri State University in Warrensburg, Missouri. She has practiced in child welfare for twenty-five years as an adoption worker, serving the special needs of waiting children; deputy director and therapist in a residential treatment facility; home-based therapist for children and families; and children's therapist in a drug and alcohol residential treatment program. Currently, she consults with public child welfare agencies to provide family-centered social services and training in the areas of family life and parenting education.

Eugene Hughley Jr. is a limited licensed psychologist by the state of Michigan, currently on sabbatical from the State of Michigan Department of Community Health. He is president of Systems for Professional Education, Consultation, Training, Research, and Utilization Management (S.P.E.C.T.R.U.M.). Through S.P.E.C.T.R.U.M. he provides dispute/conflict resolution training and mediation services to governmental and private organizations and in family conflict/ divorce settlement. His current research focus is on Copology Identification and Violence Intervention Cycle (CIVIC) as an early intervention model for preventing violence in school-age children.

George L. Jones is the associate director for Counseling and Psychological Services at Clemson University, Clemson, South Carolina. He received his doctorate in clinical psychology from Florida Institute of Technology, Melbourne, Florida. Jones is a member of the American Psychological Association, Southeastern Psychological Association, and National Association of Health Services Executives and has a special interest in teaching multicultural courses. He has given presentations at state and national professional conventions.

Kathryn Kramer was the director and research scientist of the Psychosocial Research Division of Duke-UNC Comprehensive Sickle Cell Center. She was a clinical assistant professor in the School of Social Work and an adjunct assistant professor of health behavior and health education, School of Public Health, both at the University of North Carolina at Chapel Hill. She has expertise in health and mental health. Her interests include health promotion, prevention, and treatment among diverse populations. She received her MS in Health Education and MS and PhD in Clinical Psychology from Virginia Polytechnic Institute and State University, Blacksburg, Virginia.

Brenda F. McGadney-Douglass is an associate professor in the School of Social Work and faculty associate at the Institute of Gerontology, Wayne State University, Detroit, Michigan. She earned her PhD (1992) at the School of Social Service Administration from the University of Chicago, and MSW (1975) from the University of Michigan, Ann Arbor, Michigan. Her practice and research interests include long-term care, self-care practices, health promotion, and disability prevention and intervention. Principle studies include differential utilization of adult day care, church, and family support and its effect on degree of burden and stress experienced by black and white family caregivers of elders with dementia in Chicago and Seattle; the use of a personal response system and hospital utilization among low-income elderly; health profiles of the working poor, uninsured adults in Detroit; and an examination of the impact of kwashiorkor (early childhood, near-starvation, protein malnutrition) among adult survivors in Ghana, West Africa.

Elijah Mickel is professor and director of the undergraduate social work program at Delaware State University, Dover, Delaware, where he also serves as coordinator of student affairs and program development in the School of Education and Professional Studies. Mickel, in addition to earning an MEd in adult education, is a certified reality therapist and a member of the faculty at the Institute for Reality Therapy. During the 1996 to 1997 academic year he was an American Council on Education (ACE) Fellow.

Johnetta Miner holds an MSc in Nursing from the State University of New York, Brooklyn, New York, and an MPH from Columbia University in New York City. She is currently employed as a women's health nurse practitioner at a family health center in Manhattan, New York. She is a primary care provider with her own panel of patients; health services include obstetrics and gynecology. She is the only mid-level provider at the center, along with a pediatrician and a family physician.

Valerie Montgomery-Rice is an associate professor of Medicine and division director of the Division of Obstetrics and Gynecology at the University of Kansas Medical Center, Kansas City, Kansas. Since 1994, Montgomery-Rice has been awarded nearly $1.5 million in grants for research in different areas of obstetrics and gynecology. She is a fellow of the American College of Obstetrics and Gynecology, being board certified both in obstetrics and gynecology and its subspecialty, reproductive endocrinology and infertility. Montgomery-Rice is a member of numerous professional organizations, including the American Medical Association, National Medical Association, American Medical Women's Association, and the Society of Reproductive Medicine.

Kermit B. Nash (deceased January 1998) was the principal investigator of the Psychosocial Research Division of the Duke-UNC Comprehensive Sickle Cell Center. Also, he was professor in the School of Social Work at the University of North Carolina at Chapel Hill. He was a pioneer in the area of psychosocial research in sickle cell disease. His other interests included health care management, cultural diversity in health care settings, and rural human services. He obtained his MSW from Howard University, Washington, DC, and his PhD in Clinical Administration from Union Graduate School, Union for Experimenting Colleges and Universities, Cincinnati, Ohio.

Gloria Richard-Davis is board certified in reproductive endocrinology and infertility (REI) and obstetrics and gynecology. She has over fifteen years of practice experience in women's health. Her practice offers full-service treatment for infertility, including state-of-the-art treatments and techniques. In addition, she has spent many years teaching OB-GYN residents and medical students. Her other accolades include national awards for her research in REI, publications in national peer-review journals, and presentations at national/international conferences. She is an active member of many organizations, such as American Society of Reproductive Medicine, Society for Reproductive Endocrinologists, Society for Assisted Reproductive Technologies, American College of Obstetricians and Gynecologists, American Medical Women's Association, and American Medical Association.

Regina K. Tenney is a PhD student in Social Welfare at the University of Kansas in Lawrence, Kansas. She was formerly an assistant professor at Central Missouri State University. She has been a social work practitioner for nineteen years in the areas of health care and children and family services, having worked in a maternity hospital, and served as director of an adoption and a pregnancy counseling program. Currently she is a research assistant working in the area of community-based initiatives for improving services to families and children.

Lloyd W. Whyte is currently a clinical social worker in private practice and is president of A Bright Day, Inc., providing services to the underserved population in Columbia, Missouri. Whyte earned an MSW degree from Washington University, St. Louis, Washington, in 1967, an MPA degree from the University of Dayton, Dayton, Ohio, in 1974, and an EdS degree from the University of Missouri at Kansas City in 1983.

Foreword

The full story has been documented, at last. There are significant disparities in the health status and health care outcomes between African Americans and Caucasian Americans. The health situation reflects the deeper disparity in life situations and living conditions between the two groups.

This book addresses these disparities by applying an empowerment model based on an interdisciplinary, holistic approach. In other words, poor health and poor health outcomes do not occur in a vacuum. For African Americans, these stem from bankrupt national and regional policies, nonresponsive and, at times, irresponsible social institutions, and a failure to engage families from their strengths, that is, from their positive cultural traits or characteristics.

Essentially, this book reflects a search for solutions that ensure improved health status by a multidisciplinary group of professionals. Part of the solution lies in applying a family-centered, community-based approach to African-American health care, emphasizing cultural strengths that have sustained the group since slavery. Prevention, early detection, and early intervention based on effective consumer education are essential elements in the solution.

Norge W. Jerome
Professor Emerita of Preventive Medicine
University of Kansas School of Medicine

Acknowledgments

For any project to come to fruition, several ingredients are necessary prerequisites: faith, commitment, persistence, follow-through, and creativity. Above all of these ingredients, however, are grace and self-effort. Without these two extraordinary factors, nothing truly happens. It is within this context that we wish to thank the many actors who contributed to the creation of this project.

We begin by thanking the great Creator for showering this project with grace from the very beginning; then we thank our families for their untiring support and faith in all activities that we undertake. Included in our gratitude is the University of Kansas School of Social Welfare, Lawrence, Kansas, and its support staff, especially Cheri L'Ecuyer and Marian Abegg, who provided assistance with typing the manuscript, and the University of South Carolina College of Social Work, Columbia, South Carolina.

Finally, we wish to thank our contributing authors, who worked diligently and patiently to produce drafts and final chapters. We appreciate their follow-through and professionalism. In the area of patience, we would like to extend a special thank-you to our publisher, The Haworth Press. Overall, we are grateful to time, to the people, and to the opportunity to present the challenging ideas expressed by this diverse group of scholars from across the country on this timely and very important area of African-American health in the United States of America.

Introduction

A great deal of hope and positive thinking is connected with the federal government health care initiatives for the year 2000 and beyond. The primary intent of the federal government *Healthy People 2000* is to promote health and prevent disease through changes in lifestyle and environmental factors. Its secondary intent is to accomplish this main objective through the following goals:

1. Increasing the healthy span of life for all Americans
2. Reducing health disparities among Americans
3. Achieving access to preventive services for all Americans

According to the latest report, *Healthy People 2000* demonstrates progress in more than half of its objectives. The priority areas showing the greatest progress toward meeting the objectives are heart disease, stroke, cancer, and unintentional injuries. Meanwhile, body weight has increased one-fourth to one-third for the adult population. Whereas more adults are engaged in moderate or vigorous physical activity, one-fourth of the population do not engage in any physical activity. Objectives concerned with diabetes and other chronic conditions, occupational safety and health, physical activity, mental health and mental disorders, and violence and abusive behavior show the least progress. In fact, there has been movement away from the target objectives in these areas for all populations (DHHS Releases Latest: Progress Report on Prevention).

Although people of color as a group demonstrate similar progress toward achieving improved health care as whites, they nevertheless show less progress or more movement away from the target objectives. For instance, in some areas, particularly infant mortality, the racial gap has widened. This observation is especially true for American blacks. However, some progress has been made in moving toward improved health outcomes for blacks. It is the intent of

Health Care in the Black Community: Empowerment, Knowledge, Skills, and Collectivism not only to identify the knowledge areas, skills, and forms of collectivism that black families and individuals have developed to survive and thrive in this country but also to provide an empowerment framework for supporting and extending existing strengths and resources in the black community. The proposed framework places families and communities at the center of the movement toward growth and change.

The fourteen chapters composing this book not only represent a call to action in the new millennium and beyond but an expanded awareness of current issues and future solutions. The book is divided into four parts, within which chapters are grouped according to one or more themes.

In Part I, *Health Care, Knowledge Building, and Consciousness Raising from an Empowerment Perspective: Issues and Prospects,* Logan and Freeman's chapter serves as the foundation link to the other chapters in the book. In Chapter 1, these authors propose a conceptual framework for empowering black families and communities in creating partnership for growth and change. The chapter not only delineates the framework but also defines the main concepts undergirding the approach.

Part II, *Skill Development and Health Care Issues in the Black Community: Empowerment Opportunities,* includes six chapters that address ways to strengthen black families and communities through skill building and a culturally sensitive empowerment process from both a practice and research perspective. In Chapter 2, George L. Jones discusses the usefulness of the Adequacy Model in building social competence in black families. In Chapter 3, Eugene Hughley Jr. presents his conceptualization of a practice model called Copology. The intent of the model is to serve as a tool in preventing family violence. In Chapter 4, Regina K. Tenney and M. Jenise Comer utilize a strengths-based approach to explore the lessons learned from African-American adolescent parents who have risen beyond statistics and stereotyped expectations. Implications for social work research, policy, and practice are addressed. In Chapter 5, Lloyd W. Whyte explores the relationship between compliance and public health recommendations. He prepares a psychosocial, educational, and community intervention approach for addressing low compliance with such recommendations among African Americans. Chapter 6 is written by two outstanding physicians, Valerie Montgomery-Rice and Gloria Richard-Davis, who address a consciousness-raising issue: the impact of infertility in the black community. In this chapter, the authors utilize data from a small urban-based fertility center to evaluate the fertility factors in a more than 90 percent black population. The findings suggest that the evaluation of the infertile black couple should follow the traditionally recognized evaluation. In Chapter 7, Brenda F. McGadney-Douglass provides a blueprint for future service delivery to black elderly clients. This blueprint is predicated on an expected growth spurt in this population by the year 2030. She draws implications for social work roles, skills, and barriers to providing effective services.

Part III, *Self-Healing, Collectivism, and Social Action in the Black Community: Formal and Informal Helping,* includes six chapters. These chapters are concerned with collectivism and social action that demonstrates how to bridge or integrate informal (self-help and mutual help) with formal helping in topic areas ranging from HIV/AIDS to self-healing to community rebuilding. In Chapter 8, Elijah Mickel presents a treatment approach that he describes as African-centered reality therapy. He views the approach as a viable alternative to traditional counseling approaches to prevent disequilibrium in families. In Chapter 9, Sadye L. Logan addresses the need for an expanded approach to working with inner-city families. It is the intent of the approach to help families connect with and recognize their inner strengths and to rekindle faith, hope, meaning, direction, and purpose. In Chapter 10, Johnetta Miner describes a unique project that focuses on ethnically appropriate health care interventions with African-American women. In Chapter 11, Freda Brashears explores the historical development of the black church and the role it plays in African-American culture and includes a brief outline of the theology that shapes core values and beliefs. The chapter also incorporates implications for social work practice. In Chapter 12, Edna Comer, Kathryn Kramer, and Kermit B. Nash examine data from twenty groups of parents and children with severe emotional disorders. The research shows how mutual assistance groups can be an important resource for other African-American families coping with chronic diseases. In Chapter 13, Edith M. Freeman conceptualizes an African-centered approach to community building and health promotion. Implications are drawn for social action and social change in black communities and for future research.

Part IV, *Epilogue,* includes Chapter 14. Edith M. Freeman and Sadye L. Logan surmise the status of black health care in the twenty-first century. Implications are drawn for empowerment practice, research, and policy development and implementation.

Essentially, this book reflects the authors' primary objective of providing personal and professional leadership and commitment to finding solutions that ensure quality health care for African Americans, in particular, and all Americans, in general. This book of readings embodies a community-centered approach to black health care, focused on the importance of key interpersonal connections and on the whole person, including the body, mind, and spirit, and the environment as an indispensable whole. Violence and the other seven significant risk factors of smoking, poor nutrition, alcohol and other drug abuse, mental health problems, poor reproductive health, and lack of exercise are conceptualized and addressed in this book as systemic factors that have deleterious effects on the health of black families and children. Health care, as an integrated combination of early interventions and holistic strategies, is reconceptualized in this book as community centered and culture specific because it builds on a black value system, rituals, and traditions.

PART I:
HEALTH CARE,
KNOWLEDGE BUILDING,
AND CONSCIOUSNESS RAISING
FROM AN EMPOWERMENT PERSPECTIVE:
ISSUES AND PROSPECTS

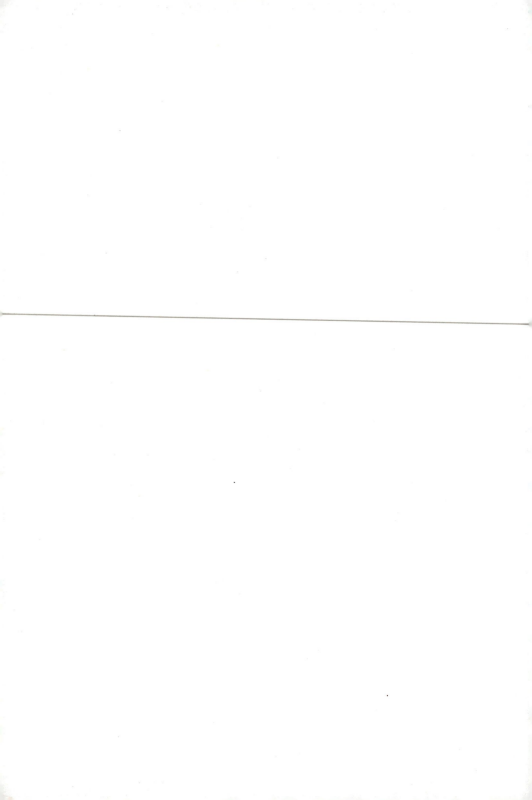

Chapter 1

An Empowerment and Health Prevention Framework for Understanding and Transforming the Health Care Outcomes of African Americans

Sadye L. Logan
Edith M. Freeman

Nearly fifteen years have passed since the Report of the Secretary's Task Force on Black and Minority Health (1986) was issued by the U.S. Department of Health and Human Services. According to this report, people of color suffered nearly 60,000 "excess deaths" annually when compared with whites. The causes of excess deaths included cancer, cardiovascular disease, stroke, diabetes, chemical dependency, homicide and accidents, and infant mortality. A national response was demonstrated in the form of the Disadvantaged Minority Health Act, enacted in 1990. The act brought to the national agenda the most persistent and serious health issues of the century. It states:

> The Congress finds that racial and ethnic minorities are disproportionately represented among individuals from disadvantaged backgrounds, [and] the health status of individuals from disadvantaged backgrounds, including racial and ethnic minorities, in the United States is significantly lower than the health status of the general populations. . . . (Disadvantaged Minority Health Improvement Act of 1990 P.L. 101-527)

This law provides a formal statutory authority for the Office of Minority Health to help remedy the toll ill health exacts from people of color—including African Americans, or blacks, as they will be called here. The act was further strengthened by Healthy People 2000, a wide-scale prevention project that established a national strategy to improve the health of all Americans. The intent of this chapter is to present an overview of the most serious and persistent health problems experienced by African Americans and to provide an empowering framework for studying these disease conditions, as well as to point a way to find solutions to these issues and concerns. Exemplars illustrating the empowering framework are presented. As part of the primary understanding of the importance of improving the health of American blacks, the health status of blacks in the United States is examined in the next section.

HEALTH STATUS OF BLACKS

An Overview of Black Health Care

It has been estimated that African Americans will constitute 16.9 percent of the U.S. population by 2050 (O'Hare, 1987). Along with this significant growth in the population are numerous challenges that mitigate against quality health care for African Americans. As indicated earlier, the health status of the U.S. population in general, and of blacks in particular, has dramatically improved in terms of life expectancy; however, statistics show that a disproportionate number of health indicators for blacks do not reflect progress or improvement. Further, this disparity has widened in some areas. Conditions of powerlessness and poverty have continued to impact the lives and health status of American blacks. These conditions have created widespread social, economic, physical, and spiritual disease in black families and communities, thereby resulting in the highest indices of morbidity and mortality in this group, and the lowest access to primary care, with little or no access to primary preventive programs.

Despite the dramatic increases in life expectancy for the U.S. population in general, the twentieth century has not been equally kind to blacks with respect to health care and related concerns. Current reports suggest that blacks still have the highest death rates among all groups. This continuing differential has been attributed, in part, to recent increases in the death rates for African-American males under age forty-five due to AIDS and homicide (National Center for Health Statistics, 1991). The disparity in death lessens with increasing age, and, after age sixty-five, the differences between blacks and whites are almost nonexistent.

Although heart disease, cancer, and cerebral vascular disease continue to be the leading causes of death among blacks, homicide is the second leading cause of death for blacks ages fifteen to forty-four and for black children under fifteen. Injuries are the third leading cause of death for black males and the primary cause of death among black children one to fourteen years of age (National Center for Health Statistics, 1991).

As alluded to earlier, HIV infection is increasingly and disproportionately affecting African Americans and other ethnic groups of color. According to a 1991 report from the Centers for Disease Control, nearly 29 percent of all AIDS cases in the United States have occurred among blacks. A special *Newsweek* report placed the AIDS deaths in 1996 among African Americans at 42 percent (Case, 1999). Black children under thirteen are also disproportionately represented among older children with AIDS. HIV/AIDS is the fourth leading cause of death for black women fifteen to forty-four years old in two metropolitan areas: New Jersey and New York.

It is also important to note that blacks have very high mortality rates for certain types of cancer with low survival rates. These cancers include oral cavity, esophageal/lung (males), female breast (under age forty), cervix/uterus, prostate, stomach, and pancreas. Other major disease conditions and risk factors for African Americans' health include diabetes, adolescent pregnancy, obesity, and drug use. Chapter 7 extends the discussion on these disease conditions and risk factors of black people.

Diabetes

Diabetes is an endocrine disorder characterized by an insufficient and/or ineffective secretion of insulin, accompanied by elevation in plasma glucose levels as well as abnormalities in lipoprotein and amino acid metabolism. Current reports suggest that non-insulin-dependent diabetes mellitus is increasing among blacks, with the higher rates occurring among overweight black women. The death rates among blacks from diabetic complications are also higher among black women, with greater degrees of complications from ocular conditions, including cataracts and glaucoma. The most common and clinically significant eye condition is retinopathy. The severity of diabetes is due to its impaired blood sugar control, renal disease, and hypertension (Klein et al., 1988; Tull, Makame, and Roseman, 1994).

Adolescent Pregnancy

Pregnancies occurring in women under twenty years of age are considered to be high-risk pregnancies. Infants born to teenage mothers tend to have a higher incidence of low birth weight (LBW) and remain at a higher risk of dying before their first birthday. Despite the decrease in the number of teen pregnancies overall, teen mothers are more likely to be black than any other ethnicity (Report of the Secretary's Task Force on Black and Minority Health, 1986). National data for 1990 suggest that nearly one-fourth of all black births were to women under the age of twenty (U.S. Department of Commerce, 1993). It follows that age-related risk factors, combined with LBW, generally give rise to high infant mortality. Recent reports, however, suggest that, although still high, infant mortality rates among blacks are decreasing (Case, 1999).

Obesity

Among black women, obesity cuts across all income levels; however, southern rural black women appear more likely to be overweight than black women from other parts of the United States. Available data suggest that people of color are more obese than whites, that the poor are more obese than the affluent, and that women are more obese than men. In addition to being a major risk factor for death, it is a risk factor for numerous physical conditions, such as complex disorders involving genetics, diet, and nondietary environmental factors (Blocker, 1994).

Drug Use

Abuse of alcohol, tobacco, and other drugs has a devastating impact on African Americans, and such abuse places them at a high risk for morbidity and mortality. This devastation may take the form of numerous drug-related health problems, criminal activities, loss of family relationships, high school dropout rates, and absence from the labor force.

According to the National Household Survey on Drug Abuse (NHSDA, 1991), marijuana is the illicit drug most often used among all racial/ethnic groups. Among African Americans, overall use was 11.2 percent, with the highest rates among those eighteen to thirty-four years of age. The lowest rate of marijuana use among blacks was among those thirty-five years and older, with midrange rates among those twelve to seventeen years old. Cocaine and psychoactive prescription drugs represented the next two most frequently used drugs among African Americans (NHSDA, 1991).

THE PROPOSED FRAMEWORK

This proposed empowerment and health promotion framework for African Americans addresses the complex nature of black health care. It describes a set of ideas that provide insight into and understanding about health and wellness and intervention needs in black communities. In this framework, empowerment refers to the process by which individuals and groups gain power, access resources, and take control over their lives (Solomon, 1990). In doing so, they can achieve their highest personal and collective aspirations and goals. Empowerment theories explicitly focus on the structural barriers that prevent people from accessing resources necessary for their health and well-being. These barriers, for example, include the effects of prolonged powerlessness on oppressed and marginalized individuals and groups, as well as the unequal distribution of wealth and power inherent in postindustrial economies. It is important to note that these assumptions about empowerment are not only concerned with the process of empowerment but also with results that produce greater access to resources and power by the disenfranchised.

Health promotion is a positive, expansive concept that came into being during the 1980s. As a health and wellness movement, it offers hope for the 30 to 40 million Americans who lack private or public health insurance coverage. It has been suggested that three areas are intrinsic to health promotion and wellness: (1) self-care, which refers to the choices individuals make to safeguard their own health, (2) mutual aid, which refers to people's joint efforts to handle health problems, and (3) a healthy environment, which refers to policy development and implementation that supports the creation of physical, social, and economic conditions conducive to healthy lifestyles. Health promotion is inclusive of good physical health, physical fitness, mental health, nutrition, family life development, stress management, racial/ethnic relations, conflict resolution and communication styles, alcohol- and drug-free lifestyles, and consumerism (Caplan and Weissberg, 1989; Hawkins and Catalano, 1992).

Health education and promotion can be operationalized through a variety of interventions and service activities. Examples of these are as follows:

1. *Awareness activities* include public service announcements, at-risk assessment, public forums, and community outreach.
2. *Knowledge building for increased personal choice* includes workshops and special dissemination of written materials on special topics.
3. *Self-care and life skills development* provide small, focused self-help groups addressing issues related to everyday problems in living (money management, culturally sensitive parenting, healthy eating, effective communication and decision making).
4. *Resource development and management* involves people and their talents, goods and services, and the proposal for new and revised service policies, procedures, and practices that support a community-centered orientation.
5. *Community building* is defined by Weil (1996) and Shaffer and Anundsen (1993) as activities, practices, and policies that support and foster positive connections among individuals, groups, organizations, neighborhoods, and functional geographic communities. The process involves residents taking ownership of,

and making decisions about, critical issues impacting their communities and addressing policy practice issues related to their quality of life.

The four health promotion activities are inherent in the fifth activity, *community building.* Gardner (1994, pp. 13-27) recommends ten ingredients for community building:

1. Wholeness—incorporating diversity
2. A reasonable base of shared values
3. Caring, trust, and teamwork
4. Effective internal communication
5. Participation
6. Affirmation
7. Links beyond the community
8. Development of young people
9. A forward view
10. Institutional arrangements for community maintenance

The empowerment framework also includes a focus on quality, prevention, and culturally competent services and recognizes that all levels of government, voluntary associations, community groups, individuals, and, most important, families must be included in shaping and improving health outcomes.

As a means of integrating the empowerment and health promotion aspects of this framework, a community-centered approach, based on a community-building/development approach, is utilized. Braithwaite and colleagues (1989) sequenced seven steps to frame this approach:

1. Learning the community
2. Learning and understanding community ecology
3. Establishing the community entry process
4. Building credibility
5. Developing a community board
6. Conducting needs assessment
7. Intervention planning

Learning the Community

It is useful to this discussion to begin with a conceptualization of community as a dynamic whole that emerges when

> [a] group of people participate in common practice; depend on one another; make decisions together; identify themselves as part of something larger than the sum of their individual relationships and commit themselves for the long term to their own, one another's and the group's well-being. (Shaffer and Anundsen, 1993, p. 10)

Within this conception, the first step, *learning the community,* may be addressed on two levels: *functional or traditional* and *conscious* strategies. On the functional level, the focus is on external tasks that support the physical or social well-being of the group and its participants. In other words, are all the basic needs being met? On the conscious level, the focus is on the group's common purpose, internal processes, and group dynamics (Shaffer and Anundsen, 1993).

Essentially, the emphasis is on the community's need for personal expression and growth experiences. Through self-examination and group inquiry, questions can be addressed, such as, Who are we? Why have we come together? How are we doing in our relationship with one another? What might help us improve? Both levels of community needs may be assessed through the process of participant observation and informal conversations.

The second step, *understanding community ecology,* involves learning about the sociocultural, physical, political, and economic levels of the community's environment. Effective ways of learning about these different levels of the community include community walks, eating in the local restaurants, visiting and observing at local social service agencies, observing at different schools, visiting local churches, and attending sporting events or concerts. Focus groups, surveys, and face-to-face interviews serve as a more formal means of assessing community structure and function.

The third step, *establishing the community entry process,* requires the identification of key informants or allies. Several authors have suggested the use of "cultural brokers," or mediators, who not only alleviate suspicion between community members and outsiders but also assist in identifying informal community leaders and formal and informal gatekeepers (Leigh, 1998). Cultural brokers are especially helpful in identifying community values, beliefs, and ways of being in the world (Logan, Freeman, and McRoy, 1990).

The fourth step, *building credibility,* not only involves the demonstration of goodwill, respect, and positive regard for the community and its members but direct involvement of the community in ownership of programs and activities.

The fifth step, *developing a community board,* involves the identification and training of community members to assume final responsibility over community-building partnerships, program planning, program development, fund development, and the development of guidelines and procedures governing all community health care initiatives.

The sixth step, *conducting needs assessment,* is an extension of the board responsibilities and is included in the training process. Community or outside consultants may be consulted concerning the technical aspects of this process.

The seventh step, *intervention planning,* is a community-centered activity with minimal input from outside consultants. The intent behind this activity is the provision of effective prevention services that is ongoing and can be replicated.

For our purposes and conceptualization of this process, we have added an eighth step, *evaluation and exist.* This is a necessary and important step in this overall process. Programs need to determine if goals are being met as well as the overall effectiveness of program activities. As program goals and objectives are achieved, health professionals and other health promoters must work to help institutionalize all community programs and provide the means for continuity and ongoing community planning, development, and implementation.

The following section presents two exemplars whose purpose is to illustrate the nature and outcome of a partnership between a community and health promoters.

COMMUNITY-BUILDING INITIATIVES

According to the *Healthy People 2000* national health objectives, health professionals should "prevent, not just treat, the diseases and conditions that result in premature death and chronic disability" (U.S. Department of Health and Human Services, 1991, p. 8). A significant number of health professionals have responded to this change by developing alliances with community groups and religious organizations. In addition to the church serving as a unique hub or a provider of social, emotional, spiritual, and material support to the black community, the black church and other religious institutions have historically been associated with health and healing. The 1990s witnessed a remarkable increase in the involvement of black churches in the promotion of health and wellness. Within this context, health promotion resulted in decreases in excess body weight, high blood pressure (hypertension), and cholesterol of black church attendees and other community members (Sutherland et al., 1992; Wist and Flack, 1990).

Similarly, black churches were responsive to program initiatives concerning drug use/abuse prevention (Sutherland et al., 1994). These researchers reported on the effectiveness of a six-church coalition in which each church health committee conducted a thorough self-assessment of drug knowledge, attitudes, and behaviors for both their adult and youth members. Additionally, these researchers, in 1991 and 1992, utilized a longitudinal design to assess drug use attitudes and behaviors in church youths. The findings suggest that the church-based drug prevention program was helpful in changing attitudes and, probably, some behaviors.

African-American churches have also proven to be effective partners in the provision of church-based mental health programs designed to support caregivers of family members with Alzheimer's disease (Appleby et al., 1987).

Overall, strong evidence exists to suggest that black churches are actively involved in health ministries (Wist and Flack, 1990; Lasater et al., 1986; Levin, 1984; Scanderett, 1993) and appear to be an effective arena for preventive services. As a powerful force in black communities, the church continues to serve as a source of strength and supports its members' behavioral changes through religious and community initiatives. Researchers and health professionals underscore the need to better understand the relationship between the black community and the black church in health utilization and promotion (Scanderett, 1994; Sutherland, Hale, and Harris, 1995).

The case studies that follow are presented as exemplars of church-based, community-centered initiatives. These examples represent health promotion programs in black communities throughout the United States. The first example was part of a larger initiative called the Health and Religion Project, which was operated by several churches and a university in Rhode Island. The second example was an outgrowth of a program involving six local churches and a university in Durham, North Carolina (Sutherland, Hale, and Harris, 1995).

Example 1: Church Site Weight Control Program

The Project Focus

It is commonly recognized that excess weight, a problem experienced by many African Americans, especially women, is a risk factor associated with cardiovascular disease. By reducing this controllable risk factor, a person's chances of cardiovascular disease are also reduced.

Program Approach and Effectiveness

This program offered weight control classes in selected churches and support sessions by trained, certified laypersons. The course consisted of eight weekly one-hour sessions, usually held in the evenings on church property. After completing the classes, support sessions were offered to those course participants who wanted to get together for mutual self-help and support. The attendance rate for the class sessions was 80 percent.

The effectiveness of the program was determined by comparing results with those from a comparison group. The comparison group did not receive the classes or the support sessions. The program helped participants lose an average of 4.19 pounds, as measured twelve months after course completion against a matched comparison group of fellow church members who did not participate who reported a .6 pound weight gain.

Entry and Implementation

The church pastor was contacted by mail by health professionals asking for an appointment. At least one health professional met with the pastor, offered a full explanation of the program, and secured the pastor's agreement to participate in the project. Pastors who agreed to participate were asked to consult the church's board for approval and to provide at least one lay member who would serve as that church's weight control leader. Most of the pastors who were approached agreed to participate.

With pastoral support, church lay members were recruited to become volunteer weight control leaders. Under the direction of the health education specialist, the volunteers' training lasted for sixteen hours over four weeks. Volunteers were also taught small learning group management techniques, and necessary administrative procedures, and were instructed on how to complete forms. In addition to being given a written examination at the completion of the training, the volunteers were given a demonstration of the standardized methods for weighing course participants.

The health professionals initiated contact with the church about participating in the program, conducted the training, and provided consultation when needed.

Example 2: Church Fitness Program

Project Focus

According to Hatch and colleagues (1986), inadequate exercise is a risk factor for cardiovascular disease. It has been shown that adequate exercise not only strengthens the heart muscle but reduces the ill effects of stress and causes a loss of excess weight.

Program Approach and Effectiveness

This program, similar to other church-based programs across the country, offered services in partnership with local organizations and service agencies. For example, this program was funded by the American Heart Association and sponsored by the University of

North Carolina, Chapel Hill. Six churches participated and contributed a total of fourteen members who became course instructors. Each instructor had to be cleared by his or her personal physician and complete forty-two hours of instruction, demonstration, and testing. Upon completion, each was awarded a certificate, participated in a graduation service, and received continuing education credit. In addition to instructional duties, each volunteer was expected to serve as an advocate for the program and for healthier lifestyles in general. The course content was drawn from cardiovascular education and aerobic exercise, and it included information on the heart, healthy nutrition, smoking cessation, weight management, and blood pressure control. Decision-making and problem-solving skills development sessions were also included. Program evaluation suggested that the health instruction improved the participants' flexibility (85 percent) and body tone (90 percent), reduced blood pressure (50 percent), and lowered their resting heart rate (40 percent).

Entry and Implementation

The entry process was planned and implemented through the Durham Ministerial Alliance. Prior to meeting with the alliance, each minister was approached by health professionals who discussed health risks faced by African Americans and the potential benefits of church-based health programs. The ministers not only suggested names for a community "oversight board" but advocated for the program within their individual churches and attended a ministerial workshop, during which the program was explained and ministers participated in an aerobic exercise session. The health professionals designed and conducted the training, consulted as needed with community representatives, and provided continuing education.

Evidence has shown that ministers and their congregations are strong supporters of improving the quality of health care in their communities (Olsen et al., 1988; Sutherland, Hale, and Harris, 1995). Scanderett (1993) has shown how, through community action, the black church can play a role in health utilization in the black community. He and many others have strongly suggested that to meet the challenge of the year 2000 health objectives, health professionals and other health promoters must have an understanding of the relationship between the African-American community and the role of the black church (Lincoln and Mamiya, 1990).

CONCLUSION

The emphasis of this discussion was on empowering African-American communities for health promotion through the development of community-centered programs and activities. Eight steps were presented to guide communities and health promoters in building communities and strong partnerships: learning the community, understanding community ecology, establishing the community entry process, building credibility, developing a community board, conducting needs assessment, intervention planning, and evaluation and exist.

Black churches have a long and rich history of helping African Americans to cope not only with everyday problems in living but with the harsher realities of living in a racist society. They are also instrumental in building linkages to limited resources. In this regard, many health care organizations have moved beyond enlisting black churches only to ensure entry into the community, to utilizing the church members in the delivery of services, to active partnerships with the churches. It is imperative that the churches, as well as other organizations, be supported in building empowering capacities for promoting health within black communities. In capitalizing on the rich resources of the black community, it would be useful to keep the long view, as is suggested in the vision of Somé (1998, p. 91):

> . . . being in community leads to a healthy sense of belonging, greater generosity, better distribution of resources and a greater awareness of the needs of the self and the other. In community, the needs of the one are the needs of the many. . . . To honor and support its members is in the self-interest of any community.

REFERENCES

Appleby, S., Kocal, J., Filinson, R., Hammond, C., Prebis, J., Ellor, J., and Enright, C. (1987). *Church-based counseling services for older persons with*

Alzheimer's disease and their families. Resources in Education (ERIC Clearinghouse). ED 2858.

Blocker, D.E. (1994). Nutrition concerns of black Americans. In I.L. Livingston (Ed.), *Handbook of black American health: The mosaic of conditions, issues, policies and prospects* (pp. 269-281). Westport, CT: Greenwood Press.

Braithwaite, R.L., Murphy, F., Lythcott, N., and Blumenthal, D.S. (1989). Community organization and development for health promotion with an urban black community: A conceptual model. *Health Education, 20*(5), 56-60.

Caplan, M.Z. and Weissberg, R.P. (1989). Promoting social competence in early adolescence: Developmental considerations. In B.H. Schneider, G. Attili, J. Nadel, and R.P. Weissberg (Eds.), *Social competence in developmental perspective* (pp. 371-385). Boston: Kluwer.

Case, E. (1999). The good news about black America (and why many blacks aren't celebrating). *Newsweek,* June 7, 28-33.

Disadvantaged Minority Health Improvement Act. P.L. 101-527 (1990).

Gardner, J.W. (1994). *Building community for leadership studies program.* Washington, DC: Independent Sector.

Hatch, J.W., Cunningham, A.C., Woods, W.W., and Snipes, F.C. (1986). The fitness through churches project: Description of a community-based cardiovascular promotion intervention. *Hygie* (3), 9-12.

Hawkins, J. and Catalano, R.F. (1992). *Communities that care: Action for drug abuse prevention.* San Francisco: Jossey-Bass.

Klein, R., Klein, B.E.K., Moss, S.E., Davis, M.D., and DeMets, D.C. (1988). Glycosyl and hemoglobin predicts the incidence and progression of diabetic retinopathy. *Journal of the American Medical Association, 260,* 2864-2871.

Lasater, T.M., Wells, B.L., Carleton, R.A., and Elder, R.A. (1986). The role of churches in disease prevention research studies. *Public Health Representative, 1*(2), 125-131.

Leigh, J.W. (1998). *Communicating for cultural competence.* Boston: Allyn and Bacon.

Levin, J.S. (1984). The role of the black church in community medicine. *Journal of National Medical Association, 75*(5), 477-483.

Lincoln, C.E. and Mamiya, L.H. (1990). The religious dimension: Toward a sociology of black churches. In C.E. Lincoln and L.H. Mamiya (Eds.), *The black church in the African American experience* (pp. 1-19). Durham, NC: Duke University Press.

Logan, S., Freeman, E., and McRoy, R. (1990). *Social work practice with black families: A culturally specific approach.* New York: Longman.

National Center for Health Statistics (1991). *Health United States 1990.* Department of Health and Human Services Publication No. (PHS) 91-1232. Hyattville, MD: Public Health Service.

NHSDA (1991). *National household survey on drug abuse: Main findings 1990.* Department of Health and Human Services Publication No. (ADM) 91-1788. Washington, DC: U.S. Department of Health and Human Services.

O'Hare, W.P. (1987). Black demographic trends in the 1980s. *Milbank Quarterly,* *65*(Supp.), 35-55.

Olsen, L., Reis, J., Murphy, L., and Gehm, H. (1988). The religious community as a partner in health care. *Journal of Community Health, 13*(4), 249-257.

Report of the Secretary's Task Force on Black and Minority Health (1986). *Executive summary.* U.S. Department of Health and Human Services Publication No. 186-620-638. 40716. Washington, DC: Government Printing Office.

Scanderett, A. (1993). The influence of religion on health behaviors of attenders of the black Baptist church. Doctoral dissertation, University of Oregon, Eugene, OR.

Scanderett, A. (1994). The black church as a participant in community health interventions. *Journal of Health Education, 25*(3), 183-185.

Shaffer, C.R. and Anundsen, K. (1993). *Creating community anywhere.* New York: Putnam Publishing Group.

Solomon, B.B. (1990). Counseling black families at inner city church sites. In H.E. Cheatham and J.B. Stewart (Eds.), *Black families: Interdisciplinary perspectives* (pp. 348-359). New Brunswick, NJ, and London: Transaction Publishers.

Somé, M.P. (1998). *The healing wisdom of Africa.* New York: Jeremy P. Tracher/ Putnam.

Sutherland, M., Barber, M., Harris, G., and Cowart, M. (1992). Health promotion in southern rural black churches: A program model. *Journal of Health Education, 23*(2), 109-111.

Sutherland, M., Hale, C.D., and Harris, G.J. (1995). Community health promotion: The church as partner. *The Journal of Primary Prevention, 76*(2), 201-216.

Sutherland, M., Harris, G., Kissinger, M., Lapping, S., Cowart, M., Warner, V., Lewis, J., and Turner, L. (1994). Church-based youth drug prevention programs in African-American communities. *Wellness Perspectives, 10*(2), 3-22.

Tull, E., Makame, M.H., and Roseman, J. (1994). Diabetes mellitus in the African American population. In I.L. Livingston (Ed.), *Handbook of black American health: The mosaic of conditions, issues, policies, and prospects* (pp. 94-109). Westport, CT: Greenwood Press.

U.S. Department of Commerce (1993). *We the American blacks.* Department of Commerce Economic and Statistics Administration, Bureau of the Census Publication #350-631. Washington, DC: U.S. Government Printing Office.

U.S. Department of Health and Human Services (1991). *Healthy people 2000: National health promotion and disease prevention objectives.* Department of Health and Human Services Publication No. (PHS) 91-50212. Washington, DC: U.S. Government Printing Office.

Weil, M.O. (1996). Community building: Building community practice. *Social Work, 41*(5), 482-499.

Wist, W.H. and Flack, J.M. (1990). A church-based cholesterol education program. *Public Health Reports, 105*(4), 381-388.

PART II:
SKILL DEVELOPMENT
AND HEALTH CARE ISSUES
IN THE BLACK COMMUNITY:
EMPOWERMENT OPPORTUNITIES

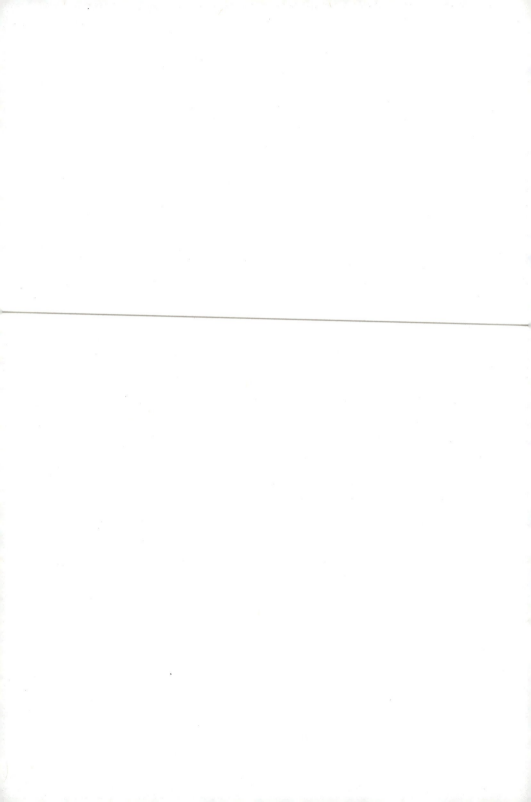

Chapter 2

Strengthening Black Families by Building Social Competence

George L. Jones

This chapter is written primarily for helping professionals and others who work with clients of diverse backgrounds, particularly blacks or African-American families. It is hoped that, through the information presented, practitioners can better provide competent assessment and treatment services to diverse families. This chapter is focused on the integration and application of knowledge and skills in assessing and strengthening social competence in black families.

The Adequacy Model, which is the focal point of this discussion, encourages practitioners to intervene with black families at multiple levels. This model is designed to empower families to be more effective in their current environment or situation. It focuses on three levels of concern: development, skills, and social competence. It is believed that a family which feels more empowered will be more effective in addressing the challenges it experiences on a daily basis.

HISTORICAL INFLUENCES

Unique Aspects of Black Family Life

Black families are unique in the within-group diversity that they present to helping professionals. The black family and black culture in general also represent a distinct racial/ethnic experience that is different from that of the majority population in the United States in a number of ways. The uniqueness of African Americans includes some of the following areas: history and ancestry in Africa, slavery, racism, and discrimination. Based on some of these historical experiences, black families have been cut off from cultural resources and strengths that helped in the socialization of their children in the past. Currently, black parents may have difficulties establishing meaningful social relationships and constructively manipulating systems that play a significant role in their lives. These difficulties can create a sense of powerlessness in problem solving that may be communicated indirectly to their children—that the parents have no control over what happens to the family.

Similar to other ethnic groups, many black children in this country reach physical adulthood before they are ready to function in adult social roles. Parents in nonnurturing environments are often significantly impacted by conditions, such as racial discrimination, that inhibit their ability to effectively guide their children through adolescence and into adulthood. Research and experience have shown that collaborative projects carried out by mental health professionals and parents can build social competence and self-esteem in high-risk black children and youths.

Barriers to Social Competence in Black Children

Research on black children displaying maladaptive behavior has often revealed perspective-taking deficits (Chandler, 1973; Little, 1978). Modeling appears to be a very important component in helping children develop perspective taking, as does the opportunity for them to learn how to correct their own behavior. The modeling of socially responsible behavior facilitates the development of social responsibility in young children, and more so if the model is seen by the child as having control over desired resources and as being concerned with the child's welfare (Elder, 1963).

Toward Social Competence

A promising approach to social competence development in black children and families is the use of racial/cultural identity development models, which help practitioners recognize within-group or individual differences in black families. These models were developed in the late 1970s as a way of better understanding some of the developmental stages that multicultural groups go through. The primary intent of these models was to help practitioners have a better frame of reference for minority groups. These models acknowledge the sociopolitical influences that shape minority identity. An important underlying assumption of the racial/cultural identity models is that they could help explain some of the issues the minority individual may be experiencing. Once there is an understanding of where the individual is in terms of developmental stages, a more accurate delineation of the dynamics becomes possible, which may result in better prescriptive treatment. A second strength of the racial/cultural identity model lies in its potential diagnostic value (Helms, 1985). Research now suggests that a minority individual's reaction to counseling, the counseling process, and the counselor is influenced by his or her cultural/racial identity and is not simply linked to minority group membership. Equipped with this powerful information, practitioners are now in a position in which they can impact black children and families in very positive ways.

THE ADEQUACY MODEL: ONE APPROACH TO COMPETENCE DEVELOPMENT

Rationale

Professionals who work with black families need to understand the strengths of black families. To be effective providers of services, they should differentiate between what is functional and what is dysfunctional in the black family. A great deal of cultural diversity exists among black families that is often overlooked or misunderstood, and practitioners need to be aware of this when serving these clients. The goal is to take these clients through processes that reduce racial/ethnic stress and lead to their maximum functioning as families in terms of social competence. Social competence is defined as the ability to form cooperative and interdependent relationships with peers and significant others in one's environment.

The Adequacy Model: Overview

The Adequacy Model is innovative, simple to apply, and designed to empower families and children. The practitioner works with most, or all, of the family members. The model is built on the premise that the family is the cornerstone of learning for children and that, as a resource, it has not been utilized as well as it could be. This model is also valuable in obtaining knowledge about what works in disadvantaged neighborhoods. Many successful individuals, such as business leaders, educators, and sports stars, have come out of impoverished environments. The model can provide very valuable information on the key characteristics of these individuals that helped them to develop social competence and self-esteem. This goal can be accomplished by exploring how they developed their problem-solving approach and how they saw the problems in their environment. This information would be invaluable in influencing the direction of public policy or in providing services to the unserved or underserved in impoverished communities.

Success of the model can be evaluated based on the development of interpersonal competence in children and adolescents. To be considered competent, behavior by a child need not be exceptional; it only needs to be adequate.

Description of the Model

The Adequacy Model is an approach to working with families and children that focuses on intervening with the client or family at multiple levels in a collaborative manner. The levels include child, parent, and practitioner. The primary goal is to empower everyone involved in the process.

In the Adequacy Model, the concept of empowering black families is emphasized and incorporated into the treatment process. Empowerment, as used in this model, is defined as

> the process whereby the therapist restructures the family to facilitate the appropriate designation and use of power within

the family system and to mobilize the family's ability to successfully interact with external systems. (Boyd-Franklin, 1989, p. 76)

Empowerment, then, consists of helping family members gain the ability to make and implement basic decisions in their own lives and the lives of their children. This may mean helping parents to take back control of their own families and to believe that they can effect important changes themselves.

A key characteristic of this model is its emphasis on collaboration. It demonstrates how traditional treatment services can be moved outside the clinic setting and applied at the community level and directly with families. A collaborative project carried out with mental health professionals and parents can build social competence and self-esteem in high-risk children and youths. The approach demonstrates how clinicians and parents can form a joint partnership aimed at enhancing the black child's social competence. For example, a collaborative project may be to help a child reduce aggressive behavior in the classroom. The Adequacy Model is designed around appropriate interventions that take into account the predominant mode of child-parent interaction in the home. Here, the children actively engage their parents concerning controls, limit setting, and dependent activities. The design of the model also takes into account developmental issues that concern learning readiness. This readiness is reflected in basic developmental tasks, such as trust, the acceptance of beginning inner and outer controls, the beginning of autonomous functioning, and, finally, the exercise of initiative.

Not unlike other models, in the Adequacy Model, the family is seen as the primary and most powerful agent of socialization of children. Parents are the initial and most enduring social contacts the child encounters. These early contacts with parents are likely to be critical in shaping children's self-concept, their expectations in interpersonal relations, and their competence in social situations.

Goals of the Adequacy Model

The goals of the Adequacy Model include the following:

1. To move services outside the practice setting and to apply them within communities and with black families, similar to the Family Preservation Model (Knitzer and Yelton, 1990)
2. To demonstrate how service providers and parents can form an effective partnership aimed at enhancing children's social competence, with the practitioner serving as a consultant to the parents in the work with their children

Appropriate Referrals for the Model

Children and families that can utilize or benefit from this model may show a wide variety of behavioral difficulties and symptomatology. Among the descriptive characteristics are short attention span, aggressiveness, and withdrawal. These children may not have developed the socialization skills necessary to establish positive peer relationships. Some of the children may have had frequent encounters with school authorities as a result of negative attention-seeking behavior.

Parental Involvement

A large number of black children are at risk, not so much as a result of neglect and lack of love or caring, but more due to a lack of social skills. Skill deficits in social competence have a tremendous negative impact on both the parents and child. Planning for collaborative work with parents to address these skill deficits and negative effects requires planning collaboratively with the parents. One of the critical aspects in planning with parents is determining what approach is considered effective. Simple and direct approaches seem to be the most effective with parents. It is important to use simple language and, in some instances, to use words frequently spoken by parents rather than long clinical terms.

Several basic assumptions regarding parental involvement in the social competence development of their children influence program planning. These assumptions include the following:

1. Parents, including socially and economically disadvantaged ones, have high educational aspirations for their children.

2. Parents' active participation is a source of stimulation and can enhance children's social competence development.
3. The family has the responsibility for maximizing the growth potential in their children.
4. Parents in disadvantaged environments may feel limited and dependent because they have been alienated by large bureaucratic systems, and they feel isolated, angry, and disappointed in themselves as parents.

When parents are involved in a process that leads to successful adjustment of their children, they will find that some of the children's needs are met. When children's needs are defined in the context of parental aspirations, parents are better able to understand and acknowledge difficulties and are more willing to take the risks involved in working with helping professionals. In the Adequacy Model, the parents are seen as professionals who are integral to the development and implementation of the treatment plan. This approach involves parents more as meaningful partners. It also increases the practitioners' sensitivity to the impact of children's and families' cultural and ethnic backgrounds on the particular issue.

Practitioner Involvement

The integral role of parents may be very threatening for some practitioners because it often requires them to take a stand or to abandon their neutrality in the work. This model requires practitioners to examine their values; their political, cultural, and religious beliefs; and their biases and to intervene accordingly. It is the practitioners' ability to convey respect for the children and parents that creates an atmosphere in which empowerment can occur.

A Solution-Focused Approach

The model assumes that patience is a characteristic that the parents and consultants will have or will be able to develop quickly. All behavior is believed to have a social purpose, and everyone involved should understand this. This will mean that an understanding of the political, religious, and cultural beliefs of the key participants must be in place. The parents and consultants must be willing to respond in a manner that may be opposite of what they would typically do. The child and family need to have a different experience than they have had in the past. By not engaging in power struggles and focusing on the child's assets and strengths, the experience is different and creates an environment that fosters change and cooperation.

It is important to understand the presenting concerns. In working with black families, the presenting concern may not be the true underlying issue. Because of their previous experiences with systems, the family may present some superficial issues, assuming that no real help is forthcoming. Practitioners, then, must be sensitive to emotions. The model assumes that emotions always support our real intentions and practitioners can focus on the underlying emotions and feelings. Our feelings are influenced by our beliefs. Honest discussions of feelings and beliefs can lead to discussions of personal feelings and behaviors. These discussions can lead to frank conversations about choices and the results of certain decisions. The conversation can then move to responsibility. It is assumed that it is in the best interest of everyone to become responsible and experience the results of their decisions.

Cooperation and collaboration are encouraged in the process of focusing on the individual's or family's assets and strengths. This is done to build self-confidence and feelings of self-worth. It is important for parents and practitioners to believe in the change process. This can help the child and the family believe that change can happen. This may be accomplished by recognizing individual worth. It is important to recognize improvements and efforts, not just accomplishments, and to give encouragement for effort or improvement. This implies a spirit of cooperation.

To optimize the impact of this model, it is important to use natural and logical consequences to motivate children to make responsible decisions. The goal is not to force individuals or families into submission. Persons convinced against their will may still have the same opinion, and no change will occur. Natural and logical consequences allow individuals to make personal decisions and learn to live with the results, eliminating hidden motives of winning and controlling. The model encourages respect for the other person as well as patience.

There are as many ways to address problems as there are adolescents and parents. The Adequacy Model is a logical problem-solving approach that can be used in a number of situations. The following case vignette presents contemporary issues often confronting black students and demonstrates how the model can be employed in helping students resolve problems in living.

The Case of the Uncool Homeboy: An Application of the Adequacy Model

Jamal is a fifteen-year-old African-American male who is in the tenth grade at an integrated high school on the outskirts of a major city. His mother works at McDonald's and his father is a part-time bus driver. Jamal is the oldest of four children. He is an above-average student and is in the college preparatory track.

As part of the educational planning process for students in this track, Jamal's counselor calls him to the office to begin discussing his college plans. The counselor observes that Jamal is unusually distant and not particularly interested in his studies or in going to college. This is surprising to the counselor, since Jamal is usually outgoing and appears to work hard in school. The counselor, who has had a good relationship with Jamal, inquires about what is troubling him.

Jamal says that he does not see the relevance of schoolwork to his life. He says that his courses are too "Eurocentric" and not relevant to him as an African American. He feels that being in classes that are predominantly white is compromising his identity as an African American.

Jamal's circle of close friends are black males in the general education track. These young men have been his friends since elementary school. The counselor found out that since beginning high school, these young men have started to treat Jamal differently. They stated that since he is in the college prep track, Jamal is not "down with the homeboys" anymore. They claim that Jamal is now acting and talking "white." According to his friends, the college prep track is for white students and

African-American students who are trying to be white. As Jamal's childhood friends have started to drift away from him, he finds it difficult to develop any close friendships with his white peers. He states that he has very little in common with the white students in his class.

The counselor consults with Jamal's parents and discovers that they, too, are concerned about his behavior. They claim that he never talks about his schoolwork anymore and that he has told them not to tell people that he is in the college prep track or to talk about his performance in school.

Analysis

It is evident that Jamal needs support to deal with the intense peer pressure he is experiencing. The counselor should be very forthright with Jamal, helping him to process his perceptions of academic achievement and view the situation from multiple levels. The counselor could point out to Jamal that achieving in school does not have to mean compromising his African-American identity, and could explore with him the historical importance of education to African Americans. Jamal could be encouraged to attain success in school as a way to enable him to perhaps become a future leader in the ongoing struggle for African-American social and economic equality or by his potential to be a role model for other young African Americans. He may also validate his experiences as a minority student in a very unfriendly system that pays very little attention to his personal needs.

By utilizing the Adequacy Model, the race of the counselor should have very little impact on the effectiveness of the intervention. It would be important for Jamal to understand the concept of being "bicultural." The counselor should explain to him that it is important to learn to "walk the walk and talk the talk" when he is in the classroom. This does not mean that he has become "white," but that he has merely learned appropriate behavior for the American macroculture. For example, a white practitioner would need to be sensitive to the issues that Jamal has presented. So when encouraging Jamal to see that when he is in African-American social and communal settings, he can freely express his blackness, the white practitioner may need to be careful not to interject his or her monolithic view of African-American attitudes and behaviors.

Generalization can also be a problem for a same-race/culture practitioner. The practitioner might consider finding a role model for Jamal. This could be an older person, perhaps an African-American college student. It would be important for Jamal to see how an African American can succeed academically and maintain his or her ethnic identity. The key emphasis is on working with the perspective of the client. Jamal will describe how he sees the problem and will explain how he feels and what he does based on his skill level. Jamal's parents can be very instrumental in this area, and the counselor can use them as models who operate daily in a bicultural world. The practitioner could utilize the parents to help maintain high academic expectations, while being sensitive to the tremendous peer pressure that Jamal must confront.

For many African-American students, changes are needed in educational practice to effectively meet their needs. Practitioners can assist parents in ensuring that content from African-American culture is included in the curriculum by working with teachers and school administrators so that students from ethnic backgrounds see their culture and its images discussed in curriculum materials. Educational equity will exist when practitioners and teachers become sensitive to cultural diversity and adapt their intervention style. When practitioners utilize the resources of parents in this process, they reinforce the parents' role and empower them.

SUMMARY AND CONCLUSION

Being an effective parent is one of the most rewarding tasks in life, and it is also one of the most challenging. The parent's job is to help the child learn to meet his or her needs without violating the needs of others and to negotiate effectively in social systems. A primary theme is the concept of responsibility, defined as the ability to fulfill one's needs. Quite often, young blacks lack the confidence to satisfactorily meet their needs. Second, they are unaware of what their real needs are and how they have misdirected their behavior to meet those needs. Finally, it is difficult for them to perceive that others have needs that are equally important. The aforementioned philosophy attempts to teach parents and black youths awareness of their needs and how to make responsible decisions toward meeting those needs.

Counselors and other helping professionals have a unique opportunity when they are asked to intervene with families in crisis. Various tools, assessment instruments, oral interviewing techniques, and current research can aid counselors in empowering clients and leading them to wholeness. By taking into account the cultural uniqueness of clients, counselors enhance rapport and are apt to be much more effective. Counselors are encouraged to see diversity in families and their clients as a characteristic that can be capitalized on for the clients' long-term benefit.

•

REFERENCES

Boyd-Franklin, N. (1989). *Black families in therapy.* New York: Guilford Press.

Chandler, M. (1973). Egocentrism and antisocial behavior: The assessment and training of social perspective-taking skills. *Developmental Psychology, 9*(3), 326-332.

Elder, G.H. (1963). Parental power legitimization and its effect on the adolescent. *Sociometry, 26*(1), 50-65.

Helms, J.E. (1985). Cultural identity in the treatment process. In P.B. Pedersen (Ed.), *Handbook of cross-cultural counseling and therapy* (pp. 212-226). Westport, CT: Greenwood Press.

Knitzer, J. and Yelton, S. (1990). Collaborations between child welfare and mental health. *Public Welfare, 1*(1), Spring, 24-33.

Little, V.L. (1978). The relationship of role-taking ability to self control in institutionalized juvenile offenders (Doctoral dissertation, Virginia Commonwealth University, 1978). *Dissertation Abstracts International, 39,* 292B. (University Microfilms No. 78-33, 701).

Chapter 3

Copology: A Contemporary Model Useful for Coping with Violence and the Related Stress in Black Families

Eugene Hughley Jr.

INTRODUCTION

A review of the literature, university courses, and professional practices suggests that a substantial deficit exists in the current knowledge, skills, and abilities regarding violence in black families. In addition, traditional theories and models which exist and which are often superimposed on black families for coping with the social, economic, mental, and health care problems of violence are inadequate. Attention to the problem of black family violence has focused primarily on the rate of violence, usually compared to whites, rather than a viable model with resolutions to black family violence. The purpose of this chapter is to fill this gap and add to the knowledge, skills, and abilities of the helping profession and black consumers by introducing copology as an alternative coping approach for identifying, understanding, reducing, managing, and preventing black family violence. This chapter includes an overview of black family violence, a working definition of coping, some professional attitudes toward black family violence, and some traditional helping approaches available to black families.

Copology is an alternative approach to addressing the issue of violence in black families. It is a contemporary, interactive, didactic, natural, and culturally sensitive model of intervention that is useful in helping black families cope with violence and its related stress. For black Americans, similar to other ethnic groups, violence is a major psycho-sociocultural-medical problem. Hence, the purpose here is to prevent violence and to promote and reinforce health, stability, and optimal daily functioning. The copology approach studies human beings, their functioning, and their process of coping with life events and the associated stress (*Contact,* 1995), such as black family violence. This intervention model consists of a user-friendly, seven-step wraparound process that includes six coping factors, twenty-one coping factor components, and an intervening evaluative step that considers three possible outcomes to appraise the effectiveness of the coping system and process. These coping factors are natural human characteristics used for physical, mental, emotional, spiritual, and social survival.

Copology has two primary goals concerning violence in black families: (1) to help black families understand themselves in relationship to the life events they face concerning violence and the associated stress, and (2) to teach black families concrete, pragmatic strategies necessary for coping with the stress of life events that may lead to violence. The latter goal helps families develop to their highest level of self-sufficiency, while fostering a sense of empowerment and safety for themselves, their community, and society. Therefore, copology is also an investment in a lifelong coping system for the self, family, community, and society at large. Once the family learns this process of coping, it can systematically face future life events that may lead to violence as well as end past ineffectual patterns of coping.

AN OVERVIEW OF BLACK FAMILY VIOLENCE

Family violence can be a catastrophic life event with extensive physical and emotional consequences for its victims. In the past, our society has devoted considerable human and economic resources to punishing and incarcerating perpetrators of violence in families. Still, little impact on the deterrence of black family violence is evident. More funds are available than ever before, but money alone cannot buy safety (Black, 1997).

In contrast, society has devoted limited human and economic resources to developing effective models useful in understanding and preventing black family violence. Given this neglect, it is not surprising that families rarely seek professional help. According to Terrell and Terrell (1984), when families do seek help, they frequently drop out of counseling after one session. This society's neglect and reactive approach to preventing and coping with violence leaves the problem inadequately addressed.

Black family violence is responsible for most homicides and premature deaths in black adults and children (Bell and Chance-Hill, 1991; Poussaint, 1972). Bell and Hughley (1984), in a retrospective phenomenologic study of 108 black subjects, found that nearly 50 percent of subjects had been victims of interpersonal violence that resulted in comas. Moreover, the Federal Bureau of Investigation (FBI) reported that 14 percent of the 20,045 homicide victims in the United States in 1990 were murdered by members of their own family (FBI, 1990).

As is the case with all types of homicide, blacks are reportedly victimized by lethal violence at the hands of family members at rates much higher than those of other racial groups in the United States (Mercy and Salzman, 1989; Plass and Straus, 1987). Plass's study (1993) on black family homicide, as a form of victimization, suggests that black family homicide is similar to nonblack patterns, only occurring at markedly higher rates. She related that partner homicide is most prevalent among blacks, accounting for about 77 percent of the total black family homicide events examined in her study.

Black boys were at higher risk for homicide victimization than girls, and children under age five have higher homicide victimization rates than do older children. Black parents fifty years of age or older were most likely to be victimized by their children and by their partners. Younger women were more likely to be victimized than men, suggesting an influence of gender on violence rates. According to Plass (1993), children are more likely to be killed by their fathers than by their mothers.

Similarly, Lockhart (1987) and Lockhart and White (1989) found in their studies that middle-class blacks experienced more violence than their nonblack counterparts. However, according to a study by Cazenave and Straus (1990), blacks have lower rates of spousal abuse than do whites, except among those earning $6,000 to $11,999 annually. Since 40 percent of their black respondents fell into this income group, this group had disproportionately higher family violence rates than whites in the study.

Jones (1993) noted that approximately 500,000 cases of black child abuse and neglect are reported annually. Imagine the number that goes unreported. Since 1985, child abuse and neglect are up 40 percent among blacks, as compared to about 20 percent for whites. The rate for blacks was 15.7 per 100 in 1985, compared with 10.3 per 100 for whites. From 1975 to 1985, the rate remained constant for blacks, whereas it decreased for whites (Landes, Siegel, and Foster, 1993). Davis (1991) postulates that the only way to effectively cope with problems of black family violence is to change social perceptions about its basic nature. Copology demonstrates an effective medium for changing such perceptions for coping with violence among black families.

A Working Definition of Coping to Effect Change in Black Family Violence

Coping, from a copological perspective in black families, is the fundamental way in which black families perceive, collect, process, and experience feelings related to information regarding life events that may lead to violence. Also, coping is how black families store, retrieve, and act on information to function within or change the environment to meet their needs. Carlson (1981) defines coping as the psychosocial process involved in responding to stress to establish balance in a person/group-environment interaction. Lazarus (1981, 1991, 1993a, 1993b) notes that cognitive appraisal, the mental act of evaluating a life event, is a crucial factor in coping effectively. The following characteristics are fundamental signals of difficulty in coping (Kim, McFarlane, and McLean, 1984):

- Statements about an inability to cope or ask for help
- Inability to meet role expectations
- Alteration in social participation
- Change in usual patterns of communication
- Verbal manipulation

Some Professional Attitudes Toward Black Family Violence

Unfortunately, few universities train professionals—social workers, psychologists, psychiatrists, and counselors—in black family violence. Consequently, few professionals have the knowledge, skills, and abilities necessary to safely guide not only themselves but black families that are in potentially violent or actual violent situations. In fact, this burden of intervention has fallen upon local police agencies who are routinely ill-equipped to deal with black family issues in a nonviolent way. Perhaps these are two of the reasons professionals have, in essence, avoided, ignored, passed over, and neglected the issue of black family violence for so many years. We can no longer pass the buck.

In personal and work situations, professionals and other helping sources cause, contribute to, treat, and prevent potentially violent and actual violent situations as black families develop emotionally. We are either a part of the solution or a part of the problem. Professionals and other helping sources who understand and are comfortable with their own sense of self and their emotions of love, fear, and anger take the time to listen to and educate black families. Such professional and helping sources can be the most useful in managing potentially violent and volatile black families. In contrast, professionals and other sources who allow personal biases, discomforts, beliefs, and values to color their intervention inadvertently allow their attitudes to dictate interactions with black families. They have not taken the time to reassess and update their own knowledge, skills, and abilities regarding violence and its relationship to black family health and daily functioning.

Often a helper's (black or nonblack) own past or current personal situation may be unresolved or not stable and free of family violence. Some helpers may view black families as inherently violent. If they dismiss issues of black family violence as irrelevant, avoid them because of fear, or attempt to take sides or place blame on either the overt or covert perpetrators or victims in the violent situation, they can be the most damaging influences on the well-being of the individual, the family, the community, and society. Atkinson, Morton, and Sue (1993), Boyd-Franklin (1989), and Helms (1993) discuss the issue as important to the helping professional's sensitivity and awareness in cultural and ethnic counseling. Professionals' cultural and ethnic sensitivity is deeply ingrained in their attitudes and is reflected in their verbal and nonverbal behavior.

Even now, universities neglect curricula on family violence and, specifically, black family violence. Students are not taught how to make an efficient, sensitive, and productive violence assessment congruent with general health. Professionals who, by choice, work toward the prevention of, and solutions for coping with, black family violence may have good intentions, but little knowledge about how to provide professional help. Allen (1978) suggested that the values of the therapist determine both the questions asked in therapy and the way the answer is received.

Inferentially, if professionals assume that problems related to black family violence will be concealed, interview style and conduct of the family assessment may cause the problem of violence to be relegated to the background. Black family members who are unable to muster the courage to initiate a discussion on violence may leave the interview with their most basic questions unanswered, and their most unfounded fears and anger unrelieved. This leaves the black family and community vulnerable to dangerous situations.

Post (1980) found that approximately 50 percent of the individuals seen by professionals report incidents of family violence. However, we do not give many of these cases appropriate attention. Many other occurrences may go unreported. If only by neglect or ignorance, we are exacerbating central concerns of black family members.

Perceptions of black family violence, the potential for violence, or history of violence as a relevant part of the total family assessment may relate more to professional attitudes and discomforts in this area than to any characteristics of family members themselves. The attitude coping factor in copology is the deeply ingrained ideas, beliefs, opinions, and values, based on information and experiences accumulated over the years about and from the self, others, black families, and violence. Attitude is the basis of one's philosophy of life on which one judges self, others, and life events, as well as how one chooses behaviors, such as black family violence or nonviolence. In copology, attitude is a built-in coping component that naturally and systematically assists in helping the counselor address his or her own culture and ethnic sensitivity, or lack thereof, while addressing the family's values, including those regarding violence.

TRADITIONAL HELPING APPROACHES AVAILABLE TO BLACK FAMILIES

Many traditional helping approaches designed to help families cope with life events exist today. Categorizing them is very inconsistent and confusing to professionals and to the public, causing much disagreement. According to many textbooks, these approaches tend to fall under four broad headings: psychodynamic, behavior/learning/cognitive, humanistic/phenomenological, and biological/trait (Menushin and Fishman, 1981). Strength exists in the diversity of these views. This diversity has stimulated further thinking in efforts to help black families cope with life events such as violence. Each approach has shown some effectiveness (Goldstein, 1994); however, people are known to improve without the use of these approaches (Eysenck, 1952). They get better, or at least stabilize, on their own, naturally, indicating that these approaches may be helpful in some cases but not essential for coping. Copology attempts to identify and utilize people's natural coping factors together, as opposed to the piecemeal eclectic approach of combining different therapies noted later. A weakness of the four traditional approaches previously identified is that none of these strategies appears to address the complete person (Heileman and Shrontz, 1983). They are fragmented, narrowly focused, and conflictual in nature (Weiten, 1994) and do not focus on the cultural context of individuals or families. No unifying approach to family violence appears to exist. It is against this background that copology evolved.

COPOLOGY: A PARADIGM SHIFT IN ADDRESSING THE ISSUE OF VIOLENCE IN BLACK FAMILIES

Copology fosters new thinking in coping with black family violence. Also, it provides an alternative method for exploring, anticipating, influencing, and explaining the nature of black families' management of themselves in relationship to their life events, such as violence and associated stress. Copology does not view traditional approaches as separate therapies, but as additional strategies in forming a comprehensive approach to coping with violence and related issues. This approach complements copology's flexible, wraparound, continuous assessment, planning, implementation, monitoring, evaluation, and modification function.

Similar to other emerging and culturally relevant theories and models of interventions, copology did not evolve from existing, established theories, systems, and models. Thus, it will likely create tension due to its impact on promoting useful change in prevailing theoretical and professional power structures, and in old, established, traditional beliefs, ideas, values, information, practices, and interests. This tension will likely meet with some resistance by professionals but will require resolution, resulting in advances in the field of coping, to the benefit of black families at risk of violence and to the benefit of society.

Copology redefines many traditional ideas as they relate to counseling black families at risk of violence. Its aim is not to criticize other approaches, but to encourage a serious reexamination of human functioning (particularly a culturally diverse perspective) by universities, professional counselors, and students of widely practiced theories, models, and their applications. As suggested earlier, it shows families effective means of collecting, processing, and examining information, as well as examining related emotions. It then shows the family how to choose, communicate, and evaluate the impact of behaviors on the self, family, community, and society. Moreover, it demonstrates specific strategies for preventing family violence as a means of coping.

Goals of the Copology Approach

Copology has two primary goals concerning violence in black families: (1) to help families understand themselves in relationship to life events that they face concerning violence and associated stress, and (2) to teach families concrete, pragmatic strategies necessary for coping with the stress of life events that may lead to violence.

Goal one involves a learning formula that must be used in the language and at an ethnic-sociocultural-economic level that the family can easily understand and apply. Sue and Sue (1977) related that premature termination of therapy may result from miscommunication between a therapist and client due to cultural variations in communication. The copology formula has five learning elements that help black families systematically assess, understand, and address violent and potentially violent life events: *Term + Definition + Function + Application = Learning*. The use of the learning formula begins with helping the black family pinpoint the term that identifies the event they have experienced. The term is then defined to explain its meaning. The definition is followed by an explanation of the purpose of the event. The function is followed by an application to demonstrate how the family experiences it. Finally, addressing all of these elements of the learning formula results in the final element, learning—that is, mastery of the life event. For example, specific to black family violence, the term *violence* is provided to identify the violent or potentially violent life event. The term itself is followed by the definition of the term for explaining violence as a deliberate, potential, or actual physically harmful act. The definition is followed by the function that helps to decide the reason for violence, such as the need to control. Further, an application follows the function, which is how the family experiences and shows violence. This informational process, in the black family's language, leads to learning, that is, mastery by the family of violent and potentially violent situations.

A basic tenet of copology helps to explain this learning formula: The degree to which the family members can communicate something about themselves and/or others, to themselves and/or others, is a good measure of the degree to which they can manage that phenomenon, for example, their emotions in relation to life events that may lead to family violence. Inversely, the degree to which the family members cannot communicate something about themselves and/or others is the degree to which they have difficulty coping with that experience (Hughley, 1992).

Goal two involves helping families learn a seven-step, wraparound, continuous, interactive framework. The framework contains six coping factors, twenty-one coping factor components, and an intervening evaluative step (see Figures 3.1 and 3.2).

Coping factors are natural human characteristics useful for physical, mental, emotional, spiritual, and social survival. *Life events,* the first coping factor group, means any situation that occurs in life, for example, black family violence. Two types exist: exogenous and

FIGURE 3.1. The Copology System: Coping Factors, Their Components, and Their Interactions

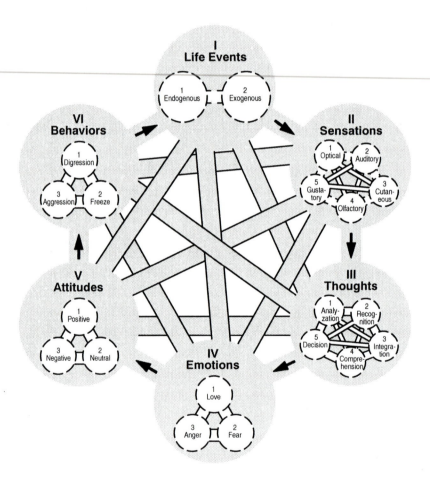

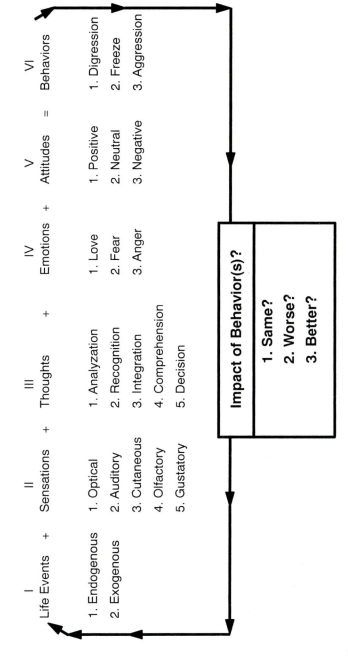

FIGURE 3.2. The Copology Process: From Life Events to the Impact of Behaviors

I		II		III		IV		V		VI
Life Events	+	Sensations	+	Thoughts	+	Emotions	+	Attitudes	=	Behaviors
1. Endogenous		1. Optical		1. Analyzation		1. Love		1. Positive		1. Digression
2. Exogenous		2. Auditory		2. Recognition		2. Fear		2. Neutral		2. Freeze
		3. Cutaneous		3. Integration		3. Anger		3. Negative		3. Aggression
		4. Olfactory		4. Comprehension						
		5. Gustatory		5. Decision						

Impact of Behavior(s)?

1. Same?
2. Worse?
3. Better?

47

endogenous, occurrences outside and inside the body, respectively. The second group, *sensations,* is the means by which families collect information about the violent life event. It consists of five coping factor components: optical, auditory, cutaneous, olfactory, and gustatory—what the family sees, hears, feels (in the physical sense), smells, and, as relevant, tastes regarding violence. When combined in their effort to collect information, they form what is commonly called an intuitive sixth sense for making inferences and predicting violence. Therefore, the sixth sense is not a true sense with a sense organ, such as the eye. This area leads to such intervention strategies as mindfulness, altered or expanded states of consciousness, existentialism, and holism, but within the copological framework. *Thoughts,* the third group, are cognitive means by which the family associates and processes the information collected about family violence through the sensations coping factor group. The relevant cognitive processes are analyzation, recognition, integration, comprehension, and decision. The fourth group, *emotions,* includes internal physiologically pleasant and unpleasant feelings relative to perceived or real gains or losses (life, health, material items, pride, etc.) based on the information collected and processed through the sensations and thoughts coping factor groups, respectively. It consists of three categories: love, fear, and anger. Other terms used for emotions are viewed as levels of intensity of emotions rather than separate emotions (Hughley, 1994; Izard, 1977; Plutchik, 1984; Tomkins, 1980). This approach simplifies emotions, gives a clear focus, and makes emotions easier to understand and to master (see Table 3.1).

Violence will not occur unless the intensity levels of fear and anger rise too high and become too painful, for example, level 4 of 7 (see Table 3.1), depending on the family's orientation for or against violence. Stress is defined as the pain of fear and anger. Carrying out the functions of emotions related to the life event experienced results in reduced intensity of emotions and stress, hence preventing violence. The fifth group, *attitudes,* are deep-rooted ideas, beliefs, and values of past information collected, accumulated, and stored in memory over the years about various life events, such as family violence. It is used to evaluate the value of new information regarding the current life event of family violence prior to making a deci-

TABLE 3.1. Copology Anatomy of Emotions

Emotions	Intensity States of Emotions						
	Mild.................Moderate........................High						
	100%...1	2	3	4	5	6	7....
Love (Relaxation)	[Like ....Happy..........Joy.....Ecstasy.....]						
Fear (Attention)	[Apprehension .... Panic.... Horror.... Terror....]						
Anger (Action)	[Annoyance ... Resentment... Hate... Rage....]						

Source: Hughley, 1992.

sion on the best course of action. It consists of positive, neutral, and negative information and is the basis of the family's philosophy on violence. Strong bias, prejudice, stereotypes, and bigotry may exist here—depending on the quality of the information about violence stored in memory. These types of attitudes may lead to discriminatory behaviors. *Behaviors,* the sixth group, are overt physiological actions chosen by the family which are designed to carry out the functions of their emotions and which impact on life events. Such actions may include violence or a more healthy action. This group consists of digression, to withdraw; freeze, do nothing; and aggression, act on the situation in some way. The two types of aggression are combative (destructive) and assertive (productive).

Finally, the intervening *evaluative step* assesses the impact or choices of behaviors on the individual and others in relationship to black family violence. Three outcomes are possible: the situation may remain the same, become worse, or improve. If the outcome does not fall within the improvement category, something has been missed (usually in the attitudes coping factor group). Hence, the copological process must be repeated until the improvement category is achieved. For continuous quality improvement, the learning formula is progressively utilized to assess and modify information and behaviors related to the family and violence.

All coping factors and their components are body based, except for the environmentally based exogenous life event. The coping factors interact with one another, linking together to form a comprehensive and flexible system with a process useful for coping.

Black families have responded enthusiastically to the copological learning formula and the seven-step framework (Hughley, 1992). A concrete sense of guidance occurs, resulting in feelings of empowerment. Through verbal and nonverbal feedback, adjustment can be noticed within the first session. The average family can learn the formula and framework in three to four sessions. Once the formula is applied and repeated, the family is prepared to utilize the Family Unit Model to alleviate violent situations.

The Family Unit Model: Use in Coping with Black Family Violence

The Family Unit Model is designed to identify and assess the dynamics of the relationships within the family that may potentiate violence, as shown in Figure 3.3. Using the model, an expedient, effective, and efficient exploration of relationships and interactions within the family and between the community and society can be accomplished. Family relationships and interactions are thoroughly examined in the context of the community and society, and specific strategies are used to resolve family issues and prevent violence. Each family member within the family unit is viewed individually and collectively in relationship to each of the other members within the family unit.

Each member is responsible for his or her own relationship with himself or herself, dually, and collectively with each of the other family members. That is, a relationship consists of only two people, and others should not become involved or interfere unless there is an issue of safety, such as abuse or neglect. People are accustomed, and traditionally taught, to become involved in others' relationships—with (sometimes) good intent. However, the outcome is often an exacerbated situation. If other family members get involved and there is no issue of safety, they disrupt communication—however faulty—between the two members, prolonging and weakening their capacity to work through issues independently in their relationship. This tends to create dependency on others for

FIGURE 3.3. The Copology Family Unit Model: Family Relationships and the Dynamics of Their Interactions Within a Community and Societal System

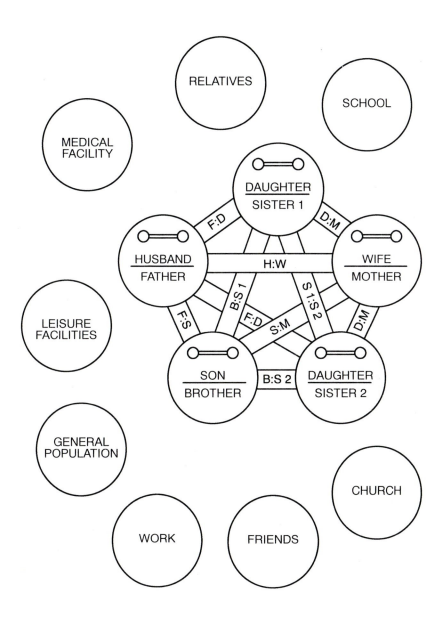

conflict resolution, leaving fertile ground for violence when the rescuer is not available.

In this approach, children are conceptualized as belonging in the family unit, but not in the marital or adult romantic relationship. A marriage or adult romantic relationship is between two people. Children sometimes interject themselves into the adult relationship. This creates a problem. Sometimes the husband (boyfriend or significant other) and wife (girlfriend or significant other) pull children into their relationship. This creates confusion and usually further disrupts the relationship, as well as the whole family unit, potentiating violence. In addition, the community does not belong in a marriage, nor do other family members, unless there is a real issue of safety.

A brief excerpt from a case session illustrates some elements of how the emotions coping factor was managed with a black family of five. This family was mandated by the courts to seek counseling for violent behavior toward one another:

> **Copologist:** Mr. X, how well do you understand your feelings?
>
> **Mr. X:** OK, pretty good, I guess.
>
> **Copologist:** When you say emotions or feelings what do you mean?
>
> **Mr. X:** When I am upset or ticked off or care about something.
>
> **Copologist:** Mrs. X, could you answer the same questions?
>
> **Mrs. X:** I don't know. Kind of like X. It's hard handling them sometimes.
>
> **Copologist:** Y (the eleven-year-old daughter), how about you?
>
> **Y:** Like when you feel good or like when you don't feel good.
>
> **Copologist:** Z (the seven-year-old daughter)?
>
> **Z:** I feel good and get upset too.
>
> **Copologist:** O (nine-year-old son)?
>
> **O:** Sad, glad, and mad. You know.
>
> **Copologist:** How many emotions/feelings do you have?

The general responses to this question by family members were "I am not sure, never thought about it, never been asked that question before": Mr. X, dozens; Mrs. X, about 6; Y, 10; Z, 6; and O, 20. In this exchange, this family demonstrated that they were having difficulty in clearly identifying, understanding, and explaining their emotions. This made it difficult for them to communicate and carry out the functions of their emotions with regard to life events they experienced, except in a hit-and-miss fashion, resulting in frustration and heightened intensity states of emotions. This increased their risk for violence. My task was clear. Through the learning formula, the copological framework, and the Family Unit Model, this family was able to identify, understand, explain, and carry out the functions of their emotions regarding themselves individually and as a family, and the life events they faced, in six sessions. Court follow-up has not revealed any further violence.

This approach has been used in a variety of clinical settings, such as the Blue Care Network Behavioral Medicine Clinic and the Child and Family Service Center of Saginaw, Michigan, and the Michigan Department of Community Health in Lansing, Michigan. From a violence perspective, it has been effective with parent/partner-to-parent/partner, child-to-child, parent-to-child, and child-to-parent problems of violence.

SUMMARY

Copology contains three essential elements for helping black families cope with violence:

1. The learning formula is designed to collect, assess, and modify the quality and quantity of information about the self, others, and life events for coping with violence.
2. The copological framework concerns the natural characteristics of human functioning that consist of coping factors: sensations, thoughts, emotions, attitudes, and behaviors. They link with the life event of violence or the life event that may lead to violence to form a systemic model and process useful for coping.

3. The Family Unit Model is used within the copological framework to assess the dynamics of relationships within the family unit relative to the community and society for coping.

The goals provide individuals, their families, service providers, and others with a culturally sensitive, alternative approach to coping. The unique culture of black families relative to violence is addressed through the attitudes coping factor. It has built-in eclecticism and creativity for use with diverse populations, including diversity in intelligence and socioeconomic levels. Its eclecticism does not come from borrowing from the different schools of thought; instead, it flexibly links different coping factors for life events, such as black family violence.

Traditional views tend to be fragmented, narrowly focused, and conflictual in nature. Copology bridges the gap between them in a complementary way to form a single and unifying process useful for coping with black family violence.

CONCLUSION

This author's research has shown that families had difficulty identifying, defining in their own language, and clarifying the functions of emotions related to themselves, their families, and the precipitating life events leading to violence. These findings are consistent with the basic tenet of the learning formula. This theme can be successfully worked through utilizing the learning formula, the copological framework, and the Family Unit Model. Copology is useful for advancing knowledge and understanding of black families. It further serves as a useful tool in prevention and intervention in coping with life events that may lead to family violence.

REFERENCES

Allen, W. (1978). The search for applicable theories of black family life. *Journal of Marriage and the Family, 40*(2), 117-130.
Atkinson, D.R., Morton, G., and Sue, D.W. (1993). *Counseling American minorities* (Fourth edition). Dubuque, IA: William C. Brown.

Bell, C. and Chance-Hill, G. (1991). Treatment of violent families. *Journal of the National Medical Association, 83*(2), 203-208.

Bell, C. and Hughley, E. (1984). The prevalence of coma in black subjects. *Journal of the National Medical Association, 77*(5), 391-395.

Black, R. (1997). Domestic violence: Why it's every woman's issue . . . and what you can do. *American Health for Women, 16,* March, 56.

Boyd-Franklin, N. (1989). *Black families in therapy.* New York: Guilford.

Carlson, C.E. (1981). Methods of coping. In N. Martin, N.B. Holt, and D. Hicks (Eds.), *Comprehensive rehabilitation nursing* (p. 2138). New York: McGraw-Hill.

Cazenave, N.A. and Straus, M.A. (1990). Race, class, network embeddedness and family violence: A search for potent support systems. In M.A. Straus and R.J. Gelles (Eds.), *Physical violence in American families* (pp. 312-340). New Brunswick, NJ: Transaction.

Contact (1995). Copology: Facilitating change for a brighter future. *Contact, 1,* January, 4.

Davis, L.V. (1991). Violence and families. *Social Work, 36,* 371-373.

Eysenck, H. (1952). The effects of psychotherapy: An evaluation. *Journal of Consulting Psychology, 16*(3), 319-324.

Federal Bureau of Investigation (1990). *Uniform crime reports for the United States.* Washington, DC: U.S. Government Printing Office.

Goldstein, E.B. (1994). *Psychology.* Pacific Grove, CA: Brooks/Cole Publishing Company.

Heileman, A. and Shrontz, F.C. (1983). *Methods of studying persons.* Paper presented at the ninety-first meeting of the American Psychological Association, August, Anaheim, CA.

Helms, J.E. (1993). I also said, "White racial identity influences white researchers." *The Counseling Psychologist, 21*(2), 213-217.

Hughley, E. (1992). *Copology: A contemporary theory and model of counseling.* Unpublished manuscript, Saginaw Valley State University, Department of Psychology, Saginaw, MI.

Hughley, E. (1994). Copology: A contemporary model useful for coping with the stress of spinal cord injury. *SCI Psychosocial Process, 11*(2), 112-116.

Izard, C.E. (1977). *Human emotions.* New York: Plenum Press.

Jones, L.C. (1993). Why are we beating our children? *Ebony,* 80-82.

Kim, M.J., McFarlane, G.K., and McLean, A.M. (Eds.) (1984). *Classifications of nursing diagnoses: Proceedings of the Fifth National Conference.* St. Louis, MO: C.V. Mosby.

Landes, B., Siegel, A., and Foster, C.D. (1993). *Domestic violence: No longer behind the curtain.* Wylie, TX: Information Plus.

Lazarus, R.S. (1981). The stress and coping paradigm. In C. Eisodorfer, D. Cohen, A. Kleinman, and P. Maxim (Eds.), *Models for clinical psychopathology* (pp. 276-281). New York: Spectrum.

Lazarus, R.S. (1991). *Emotions and adaptation.* New York: Oxford University Press.

Lazarus, R.S. (1993a). Coping theory and research: Past, present, and future. *Psychosomatic Medicine, 55*(2), 234-247.

Lazarus, R.S. (1993b). From psychological stress to the emotions: A history of a changing outlook. *Annual Review of Psychology, 44*(1), 1-21.

Lockhart, L. (1987). A reexamination of the effects of race and social class on the incidence of marital violence: A search for reliable differences. *Journal of Marriage and the Family, 49*, 603-610.

Lockhart, L. and White, B.W. (1989). Understanding marital violence in the black community. *Journal of Interpersonal Violence, 4*, 421-436.

Menushin, S. and Fishman, H.C. (1981). *Family therapy technique.* Cambridge, MA: Harvard University Press.

Mercy, J. and Salzman, L. (1989). Fatal violence among spouses in the United States, 1986-1987. *American Journal of Public Health, 79*, 595-599.

Plass, P.S. (1993). Black family homicides: Patterns in partner, parent, and child victimization, 1985-1987. *Journal of Black Studies, 23*, 515-538.

Plass, P.S. and Strauss, M.A. (1987). *Intra-family homicide in the United States: Incidence, rates, trends, and differences by region, race, and gender.* Paper presented at the Third National Family Violence Research Conference, July, Durham, NH.

Plutchik, R. (1984). Emotions: A general psychoevolutionary theory. In K. Scherer and P. Ekman (Eds.), *Approaches to emotions* (pp. 315-341). Hillsdale, NJ: Erlbaum.

Post, R.D. (1980). A preliminary report on the prevalence of domestic violence among psychiatric inpatients. *American Journal of Psychiatry, 137*, 974-975.

Poussaint, A.F. (1972). *Why blacks kill blacks.* New York: Emerson Hall.

Sue, D.W. and Sue, D. (1977). Barriers to effective cross-cultural counseling, *Journal of Counseling Psychology, 24*, 420-429.

Terrell, F. and Terrell, S. (1984). Race of counselor, client sex, cultural mistrust level, and premature termination from counseling among black clients. *Journal of Counseling Psychology, 31*, 371-375.

Tomkins, S. (1980). Affect as amplification: Some modifications in theory. In R. Plutchik and H. Kellerman (Eds.), *Emotions: Theory, research and experience* (Volume 1) (pp. 428-455). New York: Academic Press.

Weiten, W. (1994). *Psychology: Themes and variations* (Second edition). Pacific Grove, CA: Brooks/Cole Publishing Company.

Chapter 4

Early Parenthood
Among African Americans:
Support and Personal Growth Strategies

Regina K. Tenney
M. Jenise Comer

INTRODUCTION: CURRENT STATUS OF EARLY
PREGNANCY AND PARENTHOOD

The phenomenon of children having children has been a long-standing national problem in this country. Recent estimates of the problem reveal that approximately one in ten adolescent females in the United States becomes pregnant. Currently, more than 800,000 to 1 million teenage girls under the age of nineteen become pregnant each year, and approximately 500,000 give birth annually (U.S. Census Bureau, 1986; Beebe, 1997). An overwhelming majority of single teen parents, 93 percent, remain at home with their babies. Moreover, approximately 30,000 are under the age of 15, and 80 percent are unmarried at the time of pregnancy (Wallis et al., 1985). African-American adolescent females represent a disproportionate number of adolescent parents (U.S. Census Bureau, 1992).

However, one recent trend appears to bring a ray of hope to these dire statistics. Data from the National Center for Health Statistics (NCHS, 1999) reveal that the birth rate for unmarried African-American females has declined 18 percent since 1991. Reasons for the decline include fear of AIDS and other sexually transmitted diseases, reliable contraception, and a new focus on abstinence.

While the litany of negative, but realistic, images has been pervasive within academic environments, public policy debates, and contemporary media, "quiet successes" are occurring (Hurd, Moore, and Rogers, 1995). Some adolescents and young adults are quietly and methodically accomplishing their life goals in spite of becoming teen parents. For them, an early pregnancy was merely a temporary setback rather than a permanent restructuring of their lives. Content for this chapter was based on a literature review, the authors' practice experience, focused discussions with women who became parents as teens or young adults, and national illustrations. The intent of this chapter is to explore what we can learn from young African-American parents who positively changed their life trajectories following early parenthood. What barriers did they overcome? What were the informal and formal supports used in navigating through the difficult waters of being a teen parent? What were their own personal growth strategies for not becoming a stereotypical statistic?

CONSEQUENCES/BARRIERS OF EARLY PARENTHOOD

It has been well documented in the literature that having a child during adolescence has been found to interfere with opportunities for a productive and fulfilling life for African Americans (Chilman, 1988; Furstenberg, Brooks-Gunn, and Morgan, 1987; Hofferth, 1987), as well as for youths of other ethnic/racial groups. This information is presented for the primary purpose of highlighting the tremendous barriers and difficulties that young people must face when bearing children. First, such pregnancies are marked by increased health risks to both infant and mother (Felsman, Branningan, and Yellin, 1987). Such problems include less than optimal prenatal care, anemia, poor nutrition, toxemia, and miscarriage. Babies of teen mothers have a higher chance of being below normal birth weight, being born premature, or having neurological defects (Hayes, 1987; Nichols-Casebolt, 1988). Because of these and other problems, the mortality rate for these infants is 200 percent higher than that of babies born to older mothers (Bright, 1987).

Current research clearly shows young parents experience a range of challenging consequences long after the baby is born. Young mothers are less likely to finish high school than their peers who did not give birth. In 1986, 50 percent of young women with a first birth at age seventeen years or younger graduated from high school; of those who did not give birth, 88 percent graduated (Upchurch and McCarthy, 1989). Graduation rates for younger adolescents who become pregnant were less than 50 percent.

Very little focused attention has been paid to the impact of parenthood on African-American males. However, recent studies demonstrate that early parenthood limits opportunities for high school completion, college, and obtaining job skills that are required for self-sufficiency (Allen and Doherty, 1996; Children's Defense Fund, 1987; Connor, 1988; Smollar and Ooms, 1987). In spite of these barriers, several researchers have explored the relationship between family support and living with family members that helps to balance the negative effects of early adolescent childbearing (Marsiglio, 1989; Robinson, 1988; Smollar and Ooms, 1987).

For the general public, the typical face of a young parent takes on a stereotypical, even pathological image. Families formed as a result of adolescent parenthood are often characterized as uneducated, poor, black, welfare dependent, and lacking family values (Hayes, 1987; Nichols-Casebolt, 1988). Although a disproportionate number of unwed mothers are poor and uneducated, never-married mothers are found at every income level. It must be noted here that single-parent family structures "are not inherently dysfunctional, but they are particularly vulnerable because of poverty, task overload and a lack of resources. More relevant than the structure of the single parent family are the availability of other resources and the family's ways of functioning" (Carter and McGoldrick, 1999, p. 337). Billingsley (1992) eloquently demystifies the belief that most single parents are black teenagers.

Overview of Adolescent Developmental Tasks

To fully comprehend the difficult road adolescents must travel in becoming successful young parents, it would be helpful to first review ten developmental tasks of adolescence in relationship to the demands of adolescent parenthood (see Table 4.1).

TABLE 4.1. Overview of Adolescent Developmental Tasks

Developmental Tasks of Adolescence	Demand of Parenting	Personal Growth Strategies
1. To become increasingly independent and self-reliant.	Depends on age, skill level of parent, and nature and quality of support system.	Adolescents grow from resolving conflicts. Help should consist of support, supplementing, and nurturing independent care of infant.
2. To establish an identity.	Identifying what kind of person the young adult wishes to become, while balancing multiple roles.	Help parents identify personal goals, needs, and wants, while assessing strengths and limitations. Enhance self-esteem; plant seeds for success.
3. To achieve emotional maturity.	Parenting will intensify both positive and negative feelings toward responsibilities.	Label and identify feelings. Learn appropriate expression of feelings and safe coping skills.
4. To accept one's body, including changes in appearance, and develop good grooming habits.	Changes in female without damage to self-esteem. Avoidance of "badges of ability" syndrome.	Use anticipatory guidance to help young parent understand changes during and after pregnancy. Foster self-love.
5. To establish a healthy sexuality and an age-appropriate sex role.	Conflicting responsibilities may interfere with sexuality or cause feelings of jealousy or resentment.	Teach the difference between recreation, attention, love, and sex. Intervention needed for precocious sexual activity and sexualization. Learn sex education and self-respect.
6. To establish social behavior appropriate with peers and authority figures.	Parental responsibilities may interfere with social activities; conflicts with grandparents may occur.	Support to balance the need for socialization with peers and parental roles. Use journaling to monitor growth and development.
7. To acquire an ethical code that guides thinking and behavior.	Demands of parenting require constant testing of ethical and moral decision making. Effective parenting requires confidence in ability to function authoritatively as a parent.	Parenting skills training and support effective efforts. Use empowerment strategies to promote internal locus of control and build confidence.
8. To demonstrate effective problem-solving skills.	Learning to set rules for self and child. Make and enforce decisions firmly and consistently with love.	Teach critical-thinking and problem-solving skills. Guide parents while responding with empathy.

| 9. To prepare for a career. | To earn a livable, family-sustaining wage. | Educational/vocational career planning. Financial management and saving. |
| 10. To prepare for marriage and family life. | Requires self-discipline, assertive communication, and good consumer skills. Spiritual life development. | Teach assertiveness skills. Encourage spiritual growth for self and family. |

Source: Havighurst, 1972.

Task #1: To Become Increasingly Independent and Self-Reliant

An essential aspect of adolescent growth involves learning to rely less on parents or other adults for all of one's needs. According to Thompson and Peebles-Wilkins (1992), this developmental adjustment is complicated by "the young mothers' dependency on adults for norms of parenting, training, and preparation for child care, which inhibits the development of autonomy, an important task in adolescence" (p. 323). Young parents may feel an inner conflict at times between the desire for separation and independence, particularly in the decision-making process of child rearing, while simultaneously being very much dependent on their own parents for care, financial support, and guidance. A case example illustrates this point:

> One fourteen-year-old mother complained to her baby's father (also age fourteen) that she needed more than $25.00 a week to care for the child. It was time for her to plan to return to school, and she learned that she was not eligible for day care assistance, an expensive commodity for a six-week-old infant. He responded by saying, "I don't know. I'll have to ask my mother."

Task #2: To Establish an Identity

Erikson's (1968) model of psychosocial development highlights the adolescent years as the struggle over the development of an identity versus role confusion. Erikson believed answering the question "Who am I?" occurs by facing the stress of multiple roles (for example, child, student, athlete, sibling), peer relationships, puberty, changing family dynamics, and an emerging sexual identity, while integrating them into a unified, complete self. Those who fail to understand and accept their new role in the family and society may face an "identity crisis" or "role confusion." This role confusion or uncertainty might result in a young person denying, postponing, or avoiding conflicts. For the young parent, stressful issues may arise from attempting to balance the multiple roles of primary caregiver, student, employee, and dependent child. Erikson's model defines a healthy identity as one based on self-esteem, individuality, achievement, and independence.

In the area of ethnic identity development, Phinney, Lochner, and Murphy (1990) believe that "identity achievement corresponds to acceptance and internalization of one's ethnicity . . . which corresponds to better psychological adjustment and higher self-esteem" (pp. 67-68).

Task #3: To Achieve Emotional Maturity

Perhaps the most noteworthy characteristic of adolescent emotions is their unpredictability. Hormonal changes in the body are also responsible for labile mood swings, ranging from euphoria with meaningless glee and giggles to depression, acting out, or risk-taking behavior. Because of the extreme fluctuation of feelings and emotions, adults often make the mistake of belittling their importance, or even ridiculing youths. The best approach is not to trivialize their emotional struggles but to teach them to label and identify emotions and learn appropriate expressions of feelings and safe coping skills (Fay and Kline, 1990). Adolescent parents will also need parenting skill training to learn appropriate emotional responses to their children. The following scenario illustrates a potential abuse situation due to lack of emotional maturity:

> Yolanda, a single mother at sixteen, had noticed that her two-month-old baby responded with fright to loud noises. She thought it was funny to frighten him by loudly clapping her hands together just to see the "startle response." She did not know that the infant's response was due to instinct, or that she could behave in a nurturing, loving manner to lay the founda-

tion of trust, which is so necessary for the child's development and future success as an individual. She simply viewed her infant's reaction as "funny."

Young parents need direction in developing a mature level of emotional intelligence that incorporates the ability to learn from experience, adaptation skills, verbal skills, problem-solving skills, and common sense (Allen-Meares, 1995; McGowan and Kohn, 1990).

Task #4: To Accept One's Body, Including Changes in Appearance, and Develop Good Grooming Habits

The physical changes that occur during puberty have been identified by Tanner (1962) as a gradual process, usually spread over four to five years, with great variation among individuals. Tanner divided the key physical changes of adolescence (such as breast development in girls and penis and testes growth in boys) into a series of five stages that follow a predictable pattern. As we all know, physical appearance is critically important to adolescents. How they feel about themselves is often tied to how they look in comparison to others. Concerns of "Am I normal?" are commonplace. For the pregnant adolescent, anticipatory guidance regarding changes occurring before, during, and after pregnancy is essential. These discussions could focus on reactions to and perceptions of the physical changes of pregnancy and would allow young women to feel more self-confident about their appearance.

Task #5: To Establish a Healthy Sexuality and an Age-Appropriate Sex Role

Stimulated by the hormonal changes in their bodies, and fueled by the highly charged sexual environment we tolerate in American society, adolescents experience an increased interest in sexuality. To further complicate matters, adolescents are facing the onset of puberty earlier than previous generations, leaving them ill-equipped to handle the demands of such changes. Many teens are told that having sex is a sign of "manliness" or "womanhood" and will engage in sexual relations without considering whether they are actually ready to do so. National and regional research studies indicate that most adolescents engage in sex (Kansas State University, 1990). Less than 5 percent of all boys in the national survey were still virgins by age sixteen, and less than 12 percent of all girls by age seventeen (Balk, 1995).

It is clear that sexual myths, stereotypes, and incredible misinformation still prevail when adolescents do not make mature, informed decisions about their sexual behavior. Psychologist Frank Cox (1978) advises teenagers to evaluate their sexual decisions not according to simplistic, generalized beliefs but according to four different kinds of individual principles: personal, social, religious, and psychological. Adolescents should remember that their emotional and spiritual needs are at least as important as their physical urges and should play a part in every decision regarding sexual behavior. Acting in ways that harmonize with their personal values, particularly if that includes abstinence as an option, can then mark maturity.

Paying close attention to the needs of early adolescents for accurate information and good gynecological health care is advised. We would do well to introduce females to their first physical examinations between fourteen and sixteen. Having the opportunity to talk to a trusted physician who has the time and desire to advise and guide young people is critical. Unfortunately, in our current environment of managed care, the tendency to deliver health care in the shortest possible time truly does a disservice to this population. Adolescent clinics within high school settings may be a more viable alternative to educate adolescents about healthy sexuality, including abstinence, self-pleasuring, and mutual masturbation. Attention needs to be paid to the meaning of sexual behavior for young teens. Young males must be counseled to understand the financial and personal cost of fatherhood. Precocious adolescent sexual behavior should be thought of differently from adult sexual behavior. It has been the authors' practice experience that frequent sexual activity among adolescents is often the confused expression of unmet needs for attention, love, affection, and maybe even recreation. An illustration:

> A. J. is a college senior who became pregnant the first time she had sex, which occurred on the day of her mother's funeral. She was fourteen years old at the time. She believes the preg-

nancy probably saved her life, as her child gave her a reason and purpose for living.

Exploring appropriate ways to satisfy unmet emotional needs may eliminate the tendency to reduce the self to a sexual object.

Task #6: To Establish Social Behavior Appropriate with Peers and Authority Figures

Young people learn by listening to and observing others; eventually they must weigh and evaluate what they have observed and decide what to keep, what to change, and what to reject. This process of discovery is commonly known as socialization (Zastrow and Bowker, 1984) and is particularly important during adolescence, when young people are preparing to establish their own place in the world. For adolescent parents, child-rearing responsibilities frequently conflict with peer group expectations. As one fifteen-year-old mother stated, "Just hanging out with your friends on the weekends doesn't quite fit with caring for a teething baby." Support can be provided in balancing the need for age-appropriate socialization with parental roles by working out a flexible schedule of "friendship time" versus "parenting time."

Task #7: To Acquire an Ethical Code That Guides Thinking and Behavior

Ethics involves the development of a consistent value system based on what is believed to be right or wrong. Kohlberg (1969) postulated that people move through three distinct types of human morality development based on his research with men. In the first phase, morality standards primarily stem from seeking personal desires. The second phase focuses on the youth becoming aware of existing societal norms of "good" and "bad." The third phase involves moral decisions that are finally internally controlled rather than imposed by societal norms. Ethical reasoning is based on moral principles emphasizing justice, equality, and individual rights.

In contrast, Gilligan (1982) studied women and found a relationship between responsibility and commitment to others and morality.

Frequently, this involved sacrificing one's own well-being for others. Moral reasoning is based then on a web of complex, contextual relationships that focus on the needs of others, compassion, and actual consequences. To help stimulate ethical decision making, teen parents need to learn from positive role models, at the same time allowing them to learn from experience and holding them accountable for their decisions.

Task #8: To Demonstrate Effective Problem-Solving Skills

Developmentally, adolescents should be in the stage of formal operations (Piaget, 1952, 1972), which is characterized by systematic thinking, or the ability to consider competing points of view while examining an issue (Balk, 1995). To stimulate thinking and problem-solving ability, adults can help teen parents to learn from experience by giving them choices and holding them accountable for their decisions. Parents must serve as consultants, teaching teens problem-solving skills while responding with empathy rather than anger and bitter disappointment. It is important to avoid rescuing teens from their mistakes, as every problem an adult solves for them robs the adolescent of an opportunity to solve for themselves (Fay and Kline, 1990).

Task #9: To Prepare for a Career

Acquiring the ability to earn a livable wage is one of the essential characteristics of independence in young adults. For African Americans, obtaining self-sufficiency via employment and vocational opportunities can be problematic. Due in part to educational deficiencies, racism, and the changing nature of the workplace, which requires technological knowledge and skills, African Americans have been adversely affected. It is crucial to plant the seeds that, as young parents, they can still plan to accomplish short-term and long-term goals, while meeting the needs of their dependent child. Identification of individual and family needs, along with community resources (such as tutoring or mentoring), is imperative in planning future career or vocational goals.

Task #10: To Prepare for Marriage and Family Life

"It is primarily through the family that character is formed, vital roles are learned, and children are socialized for responsible participation in the larger society. Further, it is primarily through family interaction that children develop (or fail to develop) vital self-esteem, a sense of belonging, and interpersonal skills" (Hepworth, Rooney, and Larsen, 1997, p. 266). It is commonly agreed that marriage is important for six different functions: raising children, companionship, having a sustained love life (sex), safety (for women), help with housework, and financial security. In addition, the family performs essential caretaking functions, including "meeting the social, emotional, financial, educational, and health care needs" of its constituent members (Hartman, 1981, p. 10). For young African-American parents, the challenges of meeting these demands can be quite debilitating because many have not been exposed to "good enough parenting" (Collins, Jordan, and Coleman, 1999, p. 32) or are still in the process of learning these skills themselves. Furthermore, faced with the realization of limited educational and socioeconomic opportunities, many parents of adolescents may feel there is little reason to delay child rearing and marriage.

Many adolescents and young adults of all racial groups believe they have the necessary qualities to establish a family and view single parenthood as a normative event (Children's Defense Fund, 1988; McGowan and Kohn, 1990; Williams, 1991). Williams (1991) studied thirty young mothers and concluded that "[these young women do not] view themselves as having ruined their lives, and they see themselves . . . as capable of rearing children without marriage or commitment from the father" (p. 51). According to McGowan and Kohn (1990), "Those who see no future role for themselves except as mother and lover have little reason to postpone childbirth, an event commonly defined as symbolizing entry into adulthood" (p. 203). Providing realistic alternatives, opportunities, and expectations for marriage and family life are essential ingredients for success.

Review of the Literature on Social Support

Raising a child successfully at any age, whether at thirty or fifteen, requires support. According to McGowan and Kohn (1990), "it is generally agreed that social support is a multidimensional concept referring to some combination of the emotional, informational, material, and/or instrumental help potentially available, or actually provided to individuals to assist with life tasks and buffer environmental and personal stress" (p. 193). Social supports may be defined as informal supports (nuclear and external family/friends), societal resource supports (caseworker, nurse), and formal supports (minister, physician). A growing body of literature on African-American families suggests that informal social and kinship networks in the African-American community provide child rearing assistance, economic support, and emotional support that helps to mediate the potential negative consequences of early pregnancy and child rearing (Billingsley, 1992; Kost, 1997; Rubin-Stiffman and Davis, 1990; Thompson and Peebles-Wilkins, 1992). Weiss (1974) and Hepworth, Rooney, and Larsen (1997) provide a helpful listing of essential needs that can be provided through social support systems (SSS), such as attachment, membership in a network of persons who share interests and values, the opportunity to nurture others, physical care when persons cannot care for themselves, validation of personal worth, a sense of reliable alliance, and parenting guidance.

One must be clear not only in how one defines support but also in understanding or defining the *quality* of that support. According to Thompson and Peebles-Wilkins (1992), the results are mixed about social supports. It cannot be assumed that social supports have a uniformly positive impact on the overall functioning of parents. The way in which the extended family helps the young adult mother may take on different forms, creating distinct categories of support. Apfel and Seitz (1999), in Carter and McGoldrick's *The Expanded Family Life Cycle* (1999), describe four such arrangements:

1. *Parental replacement:* The grandmother takes on total responsibility for the daughter's child. In this scenario, the parent may have abdicated her role as parent.
2. *Supported primary parent:* In this situation, the young parent becomes confident in his or her abilities because he or she is allowed within a positive supportive environment to "be the parent."

3. *Apprentice mother:* The parent is actively mentored by demonstration. The young mother thus may be relegated to a position of "mother in training."
4. *Parental supplement:* This arrangement occurs when several
female family members share in the caregiving of the children.

The following case example illustrates how these arrangements
are not mutually exclusive, varying based on the needs of family
members:

> D. R. gave birth at age fourteen, while living with her mother,
> age thirty-nine; her two sisters, ages nine and seventeen; and a
> thirty-five-year-old aunt. She describes what was happening in
> her life at the time: "First, I felt left out because all my girl-
> friends were having babies. When my older sister had a baby
> at seventeen, I knew my Mom and Auntie would be there for
> me too if I had a baby. I wanted to have a baby 'cause I knew
> my boyfriend and I would make cute babies together. I knew I
> wanted to have kids some day, so why not with him? I really
> didn't know nothin' about taking care of a baby, so my mom,
> my sister, and my aunt all helped me. At times we got into it
> 'cause, you know, this is *my* baby and everybody was telling
> me what to do. Sometimes it was just easier to let somebody
> else handle it. I was able to go to school, hang out with my
> friends, 'cause my family helped me out a lot. My Auntie said
> I was 'play actin' being the mother. That really hurt. After my
> mother got breast cancer, I really had to become a full-time
> mother for the first time when my son was about thirteen
> months. Talk about hard."

This example not only illustrates the arrangement of "parental supplement and parental replacement" but also reinforces several primary reasons young women may become parents: (1) tremendous
peer pressure, (2) a corresponding belief in "motherhood inevitabil-
ity," (3) feeling comfortable in the knowledge that extended family
support will be there, and (4) early parenthood acceptance in the
family. An observation by Carter and McGoldrick (1999) clarifies
the issue of single parenthood and social support: "While there is
much political condemnation of single parent families, especially

those headed by women, it is important for social workers to realize that the structure itself is not the problem and that single parent families range across the whole spectrum from highly functional to highly dysfunctional, depending mostly on economics, and emotional, family and community connectedness" (p. 257).

Personal Growth Strategies: Characteristics Necessary for Successful Adolescent Parenthood

Qualities that are predictive of a positive transition into parenthood for adolescents and young adults are multidimensional. Recent literature on African-American families suggests that the following five characteristics are key factors: emotional maturity, family and community connectedness (social support), educational or vocational attainment, economic stability, and promotion of parenting competency (Billingsley, 1992; Rubin-Stiffman and Davis, 1990; Thompson and Peebles-Wilkins, 1992).

Emotional Maturity

Adolescents must learn to move from labile mood swings to awareness and control of feelings and behaviors. To function effectively in relationships with others, one must balance thinking and reasoning with feelings, lest the individual becomes trapped in a world of emotional reactivity (Bowen, 1976). The mature young adult will need to learn how to decrease emotional reactions and increase critical thinking as a necessary prerequisite to problem solving.

People receive little, if any, training on how to be effective partners and parents, which requires knowledge, patience, consistency, and unselfishness (Collins, Jordan, and Coleman, 1999). Social workers and other practitioners are in a unique position to assist young parents in defining the self and in learning the tools for positive emotional development and family relationships. A key focus will be to help young people learn that love is more than a feeling; it is also a decision that brings with it the responsibility to act lovingly toward others.

Family and Community Connectedness

This is also known in the literature as social support (McGowan and Kohn, 1990; Thompson and Peebles-Wilkins, 1992). According to McGowan and Kohn (1990), many authors and clinicians recognize the potential value of mobilizing natural supports to mediate the stress associated with adolescent parenting and to propose various professional interventions designed to strengthen teens' social support systems. Formal supports for young parents could include regular church participation and advisement with a minister or women's auxiliary group, and membership in social organizations (for example, National Urban League) or self-help support groups (e.g., Parents As Teachers). We would also add having a trusted family physician or nurse practitioner who becomes a trusted advisor.

Educational and Vocational Attainment

All families require fair and equal treatment from environmental systems that provide avenues for educational and vocational achievement. Historically, members of different groups have not had equal access to the same resources and systems of helping as the dominant culture (Collins, Jordan, and Coleman, 1999). Practitioners must focus on plans that help young parents complete school, obtain their GED, and identify vocational plans for the future. Vocational schools, community colleges, and universities should be considered viable options, as most schools provide child care facilities, special on-campus housing arrangements, and other supports for young families. Where young parents are ill-prepared for postsecondary education, we must help them explore career options that will meet the technological demands in the new millennium. It has been suggested that a majority of jobs in the new century have not yet been created. Being educationally prepared for this new technology will be essential. When single-parent families have adequate income and supportive resources, they can be as viable as two-parent families (Burden, 1986).

Economic Stability

Providing financially for one's family is an essential characteristic that determines the quality of life for parent and child. Problems of single-parent families are compounded by economic difficulties (Collins, Jordan, and Coleman, 1999). With the changing nature of welfare reform, young parents receiving governmental assistance will be held to a higher standard than previous recipients. The following example is illustrative of this new demand:

> A twenty-four-year-old college student states, "Determination has made it possible for me to go to school, volunteer as a requirement for public assistance, and take care of my two children. At times, the responsibilities are so great that I don't have time to sleep." She has her family to provide support and assistance, from material help to baby-sitting. She was dismayed to learn of the new eligibility requirements.

Young people receiving governmental assistance need clear, concise, and accurate information concerning eligibility guidelines and expectations. For young working parents, assistance with financial budgeting, becoming skillful consumers, obtaining quality child care resources, and transportation will be essential if they are to succeed.

Promotion of Parenting Competence

Noted child development expert Uri Bronfenbrenner (1977) encourages parents to develop confidence in their ability to parent because children will develop a sense of security from the parents' sense of confidence. It is essential that young parents learn the skill of trusting their instincts as parents but also recognize when their fund of knowledge is incomplete and deficient. As one sixteen-year-old mother in an adolescent parenting support group stated, "My mother keeps trying to tell me to put my seven-month-old on the potty to begin training her. But I learned here that she is nowhere near ready for that stage of development yet. I get support here on how to stand up to my mom in an assertive way without offending her."

The following vignette highlights the aforementioned characteristics and exemplifies the successful transition into young parenthood:

> Eve* was twenty-one and unmarried when she gave birth to her daughter, Aisha. "I had just left home and was attending school part-time while trying to discover who I was as a person. When I found out I was expecting, I wasn't happy; however, my boyfriend was very excited. Prior to becoming pregnant, I had no career goals; I had no concept of my future. Having Aisha was the best thing that happened to me. Becoming pregnant and having to be the sole provider of my child forced me to see that I was capable of so much more than I had expected of myself. Aisha's father didn't provide a consistent level of financial or emotional support. My aunt, who was of tremendous support to me, told me I could either become bitter or become better. I chose to become better.
>
> "Being a parent brought out hidden but innate characteristics I didn't even know existed. I would never have become the person I am now. I have a strong sense that my daughter and I can make it through anything."
>
> When asked to describe her strengths, Eve replied, "I am educationally focused. That came from my family background. Today, I'm a senior majoring in social work. I am persistent, determined, and I can persevere. Often young people are believed to be doomed when they become parents too early. I had something to prove. I wasn't a statistic. I had to keep going in spite of my difficulties."
>
> When asked who believed in her, Eve replied, unhesitatingly, "My aunt was there for me. She provided the emotional support I needed by saying over and over again, you can make it. Now you have to understand that this aunt had five children and her husband abandoned them, so she had been in my shoes.

---

*Ms. McGee specifically requested her name be associated with this chapter, in her ongoing efforts to be a positive role model for other young mothers. She is currently community coordinator for the Teen Pregnancy Prevention Program affiliated with the University of Missouri at Kansas City and a social work student at Central Missouri State University.

She pushed and challenged me, but it was in love. She came and got my daughter when I had a night class or I needed a break. She taught me that failure was not an option.

"My pastor was also there for me. I met with him several times during my pregnancy and after my daughter was born. He did not condemn me or make me confess my sins in front of the congregation like some black ministers do. He recommended me for a job with my current employer and helped me to gain the economic tools I needed to take care of me and my daughter. The stigma of being an unwed, black, unemployed mother is still very damaging in our society. I felt my character, my spirit, was being attacked. I confronted condescending attitudes and discriminatory treatment head on."

When asked what advice she would give formal helpers working with young parents, Eve responded, "Equip them with the tools to do better. Don't just come into my life and tell me to do better! Help me to become a critical thinker; help me to create and implement a plan of action for my life so I have the skills to do better! Also teach them self-love, self-respect, and self-esteem. Five or ten years from now I can see myself directing a program that teaches young girls from ages nine to eighteen these life skills."

In this inspiring illustration, we see a variety of characteristics exemplified: the trusted informal and formal support system in the form of her aunt and minister, who serves as mentor, coach, friend, and confidante, providing emotional support and career guidance. Most important, however, Eve exemplifies a fierce determination to succeed beyond expectations, thereby proving her detractors wrong. In addition, Ms. McGee eloquently implores social work practitioners to teach youths "the tools to do better. . . . Help me to become a critical thinker . . . to create and implement a plan of action for my life so I can have the skills to do better."

National Exemplars: Moving from Ordinary to Extraordinary

Billingsley (1992), in *Climbing Jacob's Ladder*, provides powerful illustrations of how young people can defy stereotypes through personal drive and determination, timely social support, coupled with educational or vocational achievement. The lives of Charlene Carroll, Phyllis Tucker Vinson, and Patricia Locks Schmoke are highlighted. What is striking about these examples and Eve's story, is that three of the four fell into the category of being an unwed pregnant African-American adolescent, who was still in high school, with limited opportunities for success. In addition, all but one was an AFDC (Aid to Families with Dependent Children) recipient for a period of time, using it as a bridge to economic self-sufficiency. When you examine their impressive life stories, all of the women had incorporated the five personal growth strategies for success: emotional maturity, educational or vocational goal attainment, financial stability, family/community connectedness, and parenting competence. These inspirational women realized the necessity of developing future goals, with a concomitant plan of action, using incremental steps for reaching clearly identified goals. Practitioners, health care providers, educators, and policymakers can all learn valuable lessons from these incredible "quiet success" stories.

Implications of Adolescent Parenthood in the Next Millennium

Practice Implications

Practitioners and program developers should help promote parenting knowledge and teach youths confidence in their role as parents. The role of the practitioner could be to focus on self-esteem building by nurturing both mother and father through behaviorally descriptive praise, affirmations, and by complimenting positive parenting behaviors. Young parents may need guidance on learning to enjoy their children. Parents can be taught to spend at least ten minutes of age-appropriate, positive playtime, with the primary intent being enjoyment for both parent and child. Some parents may need to work up from one minute to ten to remedy already negative parent-child relationships.

Practitioners can help alleviate social isolation and demands of parenting by identifying positive familial and community resources for support, in the form of physical assistance, guidance, material assistance, and positive recreation outlets.

The development of economic stability first begins with a strategic plan toward vocational or educational goal achievement. Using a modification of goal-setting strategies employed with BSW social work students, the authors suggest the "SMAARRT-P" criteria. Goals should be designed that are *S*pecific, *M*easurable, *A*chievable, *A*cceptable (to the client), *R*ealistic, *R*esults oriented/*T*ime limited, and *P*ositively written. Practitioners should also teach young parents the financial obligations that come with parenting. Issues of money management, prioritizing wants versus needs, saving, and becoming wise consumers are key areas of intervention. Periodic review of plans and priorities will help young parents stay focused.

Policy Implications

Teenage parents from ineffective educational systems, with minimal job training for a technological economy and inadequate role models for legitimate success, have little opportunity to transcend the cycle of poverty. To create self-sufficient families, social workers must (1) advocate for a livable minimum wage and job training legislation that sustains families above poverty level and (2) closely monitor the implementation of welfare reform (Ozawa and Kirk, 1996). The authors contend that current welfare reform policies will ultimately challenge and overwhelm young families, beyond their ability to cope. Present requirements mandate that parents work or volunteer twenty hours per week to maintain their benefits. Quality parenting could be jeopardized when these variables (limited income, work, or volunteer, school, and child-rearing responsibilities) exist. We must closely monitor the implementation of policies affecting families and advise those in positions of authority and influence. If we truly value families and are concerned about designing opportunities for success, we must become fierce advocates for our clients. The litmus test on every policy should be how it affects families, particularly our most vulnerable ones.

Federal initiatives for program development should be aimed at funding community-based programs and services aimed at building family and community connectedness, promotion of parenting competence, and economic resource development. Churches and community groups could assume a pivotal role in developing a web of services to include fatherhood forums, Rite of Passage programs for young parents, mentoring programs, and mother-to-mother ministries intended to strengthen and preserve young families. Family asset-building and microenterprise programs should be encouraged within the public and private sectors. Advocacy groups, such as the National Campaign to Prevent Teen Pregnancy, Planned Parenthood, National Urban League, and the National Fatherhood Initiative, must combine their collective resources and talents and focus them toward prevention and promotion of national support of vulnerable young families. Practitioners must also educate and support political candidates who are truly sensitive to the needs of this constituency group and their families.

Research Implications

Future research must be aimed at isolating the variables that determine "quiet successes" among male and female teen parents. Focused quantitative and qualitative research attention should be targeted on those young adults who are the exceptions. Isolating the primary keys to their achievement would provide additional clarity in this subject area. Social workers must also monitor and evaluate the effects of welfare reform to identify practice trends and family outcomes. We also encourage additional research aimed at promoting economic self-sufficiency in young adults. Continued evaluation of job-training programs is recommended.

SUMMARY AND CONCLUSION

Based on a review of the literature, the authors' practice experience, focused discussion with selected mothers, and reviews of accomplished women who have achieved success, a conclusion was reached. The authors support the views of others (Billingsley, 1992; Hurd, Moore, and Rogers, 1995) who suggest that single parenthood need not be the death knell for young people. Although early parenthood poses difficult and imposing challenges, "quiet successes" can, and do, occur. Even single parents without life goals have the capacity to respond to unplanned parenthood as a transformative process. For some young adults, parenthood acts as a catalyst for setting and accomplishing life goals. Successful parenting can occur with a combination of resources, social supports, opportunity, and a high degree of personal motivation.

The ability to plan, prioritize, persevere, and pray are repeatedly seen as strategies that transcend the negative expectations so often prescribed in the literature. Perhaps teen pregnancy and parenthood, as they have been studied, are not the real problem, but a symptom of larger societal problems—namely, poverty, emotional alienation, and/or despair. Sex and unplanned pregnancy may simply be the way young people have coped with this malaise in an environment that is unable to teach goal-setting and effective problem-solving skills, predicated on an internal locus of control. Empowerment, education, career guidance, and support make it possible for young parents to master the tasks of adolescent development and to develop the growth strategies necessary to achieve life goals.

REFERENCES

Allen, W. and Doherty, W. (1996). The responsibilities of fatherhood as perceived by African American teenage fathers. *Families in Society: The Journal of Contemporary Human Services, 77*(3), 142-155.

Allen-Meares, P. (1995). *Social work with children and adolescents.* White Plains, NY: Longman.

Apfel, N. and Seitz, V. (1999). In B. Carter and M. McGoldrick (Eds.), *The expanded family life cycle: Individual, family and social perspective* (Third edition) (p. 229). Needham Heights, MA: Allyn and Bacon.

Balk, D. (1995). *Adolescent development: Early through late adolescence.* Pacific Grove, CA: Brooks/Cole.

Beebe, L. (1997). Adolescent pregnancy. Social work speaks. *NASW olicy Statements* (Fourth edition) (pp. 8-11). Washington, DC: NASW Press.

Billingsley, A. (1992). *Climbing Jacob's ladder: The enduring legacy of African-American families* (pp. 335-339). New York: Simon and Schuster.

Bowen, M. (1976). Theory in the practice of psychotherapy. In P.J. Guerin (Ed.), *Family therapy: Theory and practice* (pp. 42-90). New York: Gardener.

Bright, P. (1987). Adolescent pregnancy and loss. *Maternal-Child Nursing Journal, 16,* 1-12.

Bronfenbrenner, U. (1977). The changing American family. In E.M. Hetherington and R.D. Parke (Eds.), *Contemporary readings in child psychology* (pp. 46-68). New York: McGraw-Hill.

Burden, D. (1986). Single parents and the work setting: The impact of multiple jobs and home life responsibilities. *Family Relations, 35,* 37-43.

Carter, B. and McGoldrick, M. (1999). *The expanded family life cycle: Individual, family and social perspective* (Third edition) (p. 257). Needham Heights, MA: Allyn and Bacon.

Children's Defense Fund (1987). *Adolescent pregnancy: An anatomy of a social problem in search of comprehensive solutions.* Washington, DC: Author.

Children's Defense Fund (1988). *A children's defense budget, 1989.* Washington, DC: Author.

Children's Defense Fund (1989). *A vision for America's future.* Washington, DC: Author.

Chilman, C.S. (1988). Never-married, single adolescent parents. In C.S. Chilman, E.W. Nunnally, and F.M. Cox (Eds.), *Variant family forms.* Newbury Park, CA: Sage.

Collins, D., Jordan, C., and Coleman, H. (1999). *An introduction to family social work* (pp. 32, 35, 77). Itasca, IL: F.E. Peacock.

Connor, M. (1988). Teenage fatherhood: Issues confronting young black males. In J.T. Gibbs (Ed.), *Young, black and male in America: An endangered species.* Dover, MA: Auburn House.

Cox, F. (1978). *Human intimacy: Marriage, the family, and its meaning.* New York: West.

Erikson, E. (1968). *Identity: Youth and crisis.* New York: Norton.

Fay, J. and Kline, F. (1990). *Parenting with love and logic.* Colorado Springs, CO: Pinon Press.

Felsman, D., Branningan, G., and Yellin, P. (1987). Control theory in dealing with adolescent sexuality and pregnancy. *Journal of Sex Education and Therapy, 13*(1), 15-16.

Furstenberg, F.F. Jr., Brooks-Gunn, J., and Morgan, P. (1987). *Adolescent mothers in later life.* New York: Cambridge University Press.

Gilligan, C. (1982). *In a different voice: Psychological theory and women's development.* Cambridge, MA: Harvard University Press.

Hartman, A. (1981). The family: A central focus for practice. *Social Work, 26,* 7-13.

Havighurst, R. (1972). *Developmental tasks and education.* New York: Longman Inc.

Hayes, C.D. (Ed.) (1987). *Risking the future: Adolescent sexuality, pregnancy and childbearing* (Volume 1). Washington, DC: National Research Council.

Hepworth, D., Rooney, R., and Larsen, J. (1997). *Direct social work practice: Theory and skills* (Fifth edition). Pacific Grove, CA: Brooks/Cole.

Hofferth, S. (1987). Social and economic consequences of teenage parenthood. In S. Hofferth and C. Hayes (Eds.), *Risking the future* (Volume 2) (pp. 352-375). Washington, DC: National Academy Press.

Hurd, E., Moore, C., and Rogers, R. (1995). Quiet success: Parenting strengths among African Americans. *Families in Society, 76*(7), 434-443.

Kansas State University (1990). *Relationships and sexual attitudes: An assessment of student parent communication, knowledge and behavior.* Manhattan,

KS: Kansas State University, Department of Human Development and Family Studies.

Kohlberg, L. (1969). *Stages in the development of moral thought and action.* New York: Holt, Rinehart and Winston.

Kost, K.A. (1997). The effects of support on the economic well-being of young fathers. *Families in Society, 78*(4), 370-382.

Marsiglio, J.K. (1989). Adolescent males' pregnancy resolution preferences and family formation intentions. *Journal of Adolescent Research, 4*(3), 214-237.

McGowan, B. and Kohn, A. (1990). Support and teen pregnancy in the inner city. In A. Rubin-Stiffman and L. Davis (Eds). *Ethnic issues in adolescent mental health* (pp. 189-207). Newbury Park, CA: Sage.

National Center for Health Statistics (NCHS). (1999). *Health—United States, 1999.* Washington, DC: U.S. Department of Health and Human Services.

Nichols-Casebolt, A.M. (1988). Black families headed by single mothers: Growing numbers and increasing poverty. *Social Work, 33*(5), 306-313.

Ozawa, M. and Kirk, S. (1996). Welfare Reform (Editorial), Personal Responsibility and Work Opportunity Reconciliation Act, P.L. 104-1931. *Social Work Research, 20*(4), 194-195.

Phinney, J., Lochner, B., and Murphy, R. (1990). Ethnic identity development and psychological adjustment in adolescence. In A. Rubin-Stiffman and L. Davis (Eds.), *Ethnic issues in adolescent mental health* (pp. 53-72). Newbury Park, CA: Sage.

Piaget, J. (1952). *The origins of intelligence in children.* New York: International Universities Press.

Piaget, J. (1972). Intellectual development from adolescence to adulthood. *Human Development, 15*(2), 1-12.

Robinson, B. (1988). *Teenage fathers.* Lexington, MA: Lexington Books.

Rubin-Stiffman, A. and Davis, L.E. (Eds.) (1990). *Ethnic issues in adolescent mental health.* Newbury Park, CA: Sage.

Smollar, J. and Ooms, T. (1987). *Young unwed fathers: Research review, policy dilemmas and options.* Washington, DC: Catholic University of America.

Tanner, J.M. (1962). *Growth at adolescence* (Second edition). Oxford: Blackwell.

Thompson, M.S. and Peebles-Wilkins, W. (1992). The impact of formal, informal and societal support networks on the psychological well-being of black adolescent mothers. *Social Work, 37*(4), 322-328.

U.S. Census Bureau (1986). *Statistical abstracts of the United States.* Washington, DC: U.S. Government Printing Office.

U.S. Census Bureau (1992). *Statistical abstracts of the United States.* Washington, DC: U.S. Government Printing Office.

Upchurch, D.M. and McCarthy, J. (1989). Adolescent childbearing and high school completion in the 1980's: Have things changed? *Family Planning Perspectives, 21*(5), 199-202.

Wallis, C., Booth, C., Leutka, M., and Taylor, E. (1985). Children having children. *Time, 126*(3), December 9, 78-90.

Weiss, R. (1974). The provisions of social relationships. In L. Rubin (Ed.), *Doing unto others* (pp. 17-26). Englewood Cliffs, NJ: Prentice-Hall.

Williams, C.W. (1991). *Black teenage mothers: Pregnancy and child rearing from their perspective.* Lexington, MA: Lexington Books.

Zastrow, C. and Bowker, L. (1984). *Social problems.* Chicago: Nelson-Hall.

Chapter 5

Promoting Health Prevention Programs and Medical Compliance: An Expanded Conceptual Model

Lloyd W. Whyte

OVERVIEW OF THE COMPLIANCE PROBLEM

Despite the vast increase in health expenditures and considerable advances in health care technology during the past decade, there has not been a corresponding increase in many of the nation's health statistics. Although it may be evident that the quality of health care has been remarkably improved in the past two decades, it is general knowledge that the nation continues to experience high infant mortality rates and unacceptably high rates of preventable illnesses, for example, certain cancers, tuberculosis, early childhood diseases, AIDS, and other sexually transmitted diseases (Greenburg and Schneider, 1995).

It is well known that African Americans have a higher incidence of hypertension. About 39 percent of all adult black females and 38 percent of all adult black males suffer from high blood pressure. Hypertension is found almost twice as often in blacks as it is in whites; it begins at an earlier age, is often more severe, and results in a higher death rate at a younger age. According to the American Heart Association, blacks have a 60 percent greater risk of death and disability from stroke and coronary disease than whites because of high blood pressure. Although many factors may play a part in why this illness is more prevalent in the black population, it is no less true that hypertension is arguably a controllable and/or preventable disease (White, 1994). In addition, African-American children are more than twice as likely as white children to be born prematurely, have low birth weight, and die in the first year of life (White, 1994).

Prevention of such health problems may impact drug addiction and violence, especially that which affects the black population, resulting in huge costs in terms of lost lives, lost productivity, and broken families. The general appeal has been for more prevention and treatment. Various violence prevention programs have met with success in several sites in cities such as Omaha, Detroit, and Los Angeles, where community educational, peer counseling, and life skills training programs have been implemented. Politicians are beginning to listen to the notion of prevention in some respects by funding these community programs (Prothrow-Stith, 1995). Largely, however, the basic approach to reduce illness has been to educate the target population through doctor-to-patient advice about how to properly take medication. Children and teens are often reached in the classroom with information about drugs and sex.

It is argued here, however, that these types of educational preventive efforts have *not* worked and that the reason lies in our *not* having followed what the research tells us about compliance. This chapter will deal generally with various aspects of medical compliance and those factors which influence compliance and prevention. An attempt will be made to indicate how these issues pertain importantly to African Americans. It is the purpose here to review these issues and to offer some interventions or strategies that may promote health prevention and/or increase compliance.

ARE WE MISSING THE MARK?

The past two decades have seen the development of highly effective drug therapies for various types of illness. Medical knowledge is abundant regarding lifestyle factors such as immunizations, medications, diet, exercise, smoking, stress, and other preventive measures that are most conducive to good health. In fact, the entire fitness industry has exploded as a result of such findings, and the public is saturated daily with advertisements in television, radio, and print media about ways to quit smoking, get more exercise, and relieve stress.

However, research evidence indicates that the degree to which individuals follow medical advice or recommendations is alarmingly low (Donovan and Blake, 1992). Consider, for example, the literature in this area, which reveals that approximately 30 to 35 percent of patients fail to follow their physician's recommendations (Agras, 1989; Becker and Maiman, 1975; Cohen, 1979; Cramer and Spilker, 1991; Gerber and Nehemkis, 1986; Haynes, Taylor, and Sackett, 1979; Marston, 1970; Trick, 1993).

Adherence to physician instructions is even lower in low-income clinic populations where noncompliance is frequently reported at greater than 60 percent (Becker and Maiman, 1975). When recommendations are for preventive measures, and/or patients are without symptoms, and/or the prescribed regimen is long term (such as those related to hypertension), only about half of the patients are usually compliant (Cohen, 1979; Cramer and Spilker, 1991). Zongas, Barr, and Barsky (1991) studied patient compliance with follow-up appointments and prescribed medications from a walk-in clinic dealing with acute minor medical problems. Results indicated that only about 40 percent of patients took more than 75 percent of the prescribed medication, and approximately 25 percent of patients did not get the prescription filled. Fewer than 50 percent of those individuals scheduled with follow-up appointments actually kept them. Similar noncompliance rates have been found consistent with these results in regard to patients dropping out of psychotherapy (Baekeland and Lundwall, 1975).

These studies reveal that the major problem in health care today is not the inadequacy of therapeutic medications, medical technology, or quality health care. The problem is instead that we are not meeting the potential for improving the health of the American population, specifically the African-American population, by improving, in part, what people do and do not do for themselves, by promoting health prevention programs, and by increasing medical compliance.

Improving Compliance: An Overview

Although it is believed that genetics plays an important role in hypertension among blacks, preventing and controlling debilitating hypertension is related to several factors, not the least of which may be following the prescribed diet, getting sufficient exercise, and, when diagnosed, taking the prescribed medication on a regular basis. Health care professionals, including public health personnel as well as health educators, can play an important role in directing various educational or behavioral interventions that impact upon this illness, as well as others.

Promoting and Improving Compliance

A considerable amount of literature focuses on educational and/ or behavioral strategies to improve compliance (Haynes, Taylor, and Sackett, 1979). Adherence and/or compliance are defined as the extent to which the patient behaves in a manner prescribed by the health care provider. This may include taking medications as prescribed, following medical or directive counseling advice or recommendations, and/or lifestyle behavioral changes, such as diet or the initiation of family planning.

Various educational and/or behavioral strategies found to improve adherence or compliance have been well documented in the literature by a multitude of studies. These have proved fruitful in providing some guidance to health care providers, educators, and counselors.

Green (1979), in reviewing many studies, discerned the following principles:

1. Information given to patients that is brief and concise is more likely to be remembered.
2. Patients will remember more information if it is summarized and clearly categorized.
3. Recall is enhanced by following a "primary principle"; that is, more is retained of the first information presented than of information presented later in the same communication.
4. The packaging of patient educational literature should be at a level of reading consistent with the patient's ability.
5. Information may be recalled and followed more often when it is written and repeated.
6. The more specific the instruction, the higher the likelihood that the instructions will be followed.

Some of the early literature revealed other similar principles:

1. "Compliance is more likely to occur if the practitioner elicits from the client an overt indication of intent to perform" the desired action (p. 190).
2. "Compliance is more likely to occur if the practitioner can provide direct training or model the desired performance" (p. 191).
3. "Compliance is likely to be enhanced if the desired performance or behavior is met with positive consequences for the patient" (Levy and Carter, 1976, p. 191).

Other helpful strategies in improving compliance have been reviewed by Dunbar, Marshall, and Hovell (1979). These include such behavioral/educational approaches as the following:

1. Reminders or cueing, for example, sending a notice of a clinic appointment a few days prior to the scheduled visit
2. Tailoring, for example, fitting the prescribed regimen and intervention strategies to the particular characteristics of the patient.
3. Contracting
4. Graduated regimen implementation
5. Self-monitoring, that is, observing and recording one's own behavior.

Reinforcements are also helpful. For example, Morisky (1990) developed an incentive scheme to reward health behaviors (adherence to antituberculosis drug regimens) and found that those who received the incentive were significantly more likely to continue with treatment and to take their medication as prescribed.

Understanding Factors That Influence Compliance

Educational/behavioral change agents interested in improving adherence to therapeutic regimens must begin with an understanding of the multitude of factors considered to influence compliance behavior. As early as 1979, Haynes, Taylor, and Sackett compiled well over a thousand articles, including research studies, conceptual models, literature reviews, and so on, that concern this topic. This research has looked at the influence of characteristics, attitudes, and beliefs of the patient; characteristics of the treatment regimen; the physician-patient interaction; and the influence of social support, to name only a few of the best studies.

Many studies of patient psychological variables have also failed to find a positive association between personality characteristics and compliance. Studies have also shown that, in general, the severity of the illness, prior hospitalization, and cost of care are unrelated to compliance. Perhaps more remarkable, especially for those interested in educational-type interventions, are the many studies indicating little or no association between compliance and knowledge about one's illness or medical regimen (Haynes, Taylor, and Sackett, 1979).

The most consistent predictors of compliance are patients' beliefs about their illness, certain psychosocial interaction factors, and "locus of control." It might be said that "locus of control" relates to the degree to which individuals feel they have some control over their lives, destinies, and environments. This also seems to involve the concept of self-image. One may take a look at this factor in relation to the previously mentioned "preventable" or "controllable" African-American problems of hypertension and infant mortality.

Certainly, African-American males may have feelings of low self-esteem, may feel unable to control their lives if they are unable to obtain a decent job, may have grown up without a father figure, and may have faced the countless stressors of being an African-American male. The young black female may also have problems with self-esteem, feeling that she is unable to chart her own course for many of the same reasons. Both black males and black females may grow up feeling as though they lack a "sense of choice." Indeed, it is likely that the emphasis on black pride and identification, beginning in the 1960s, is related to self-image and a feeling that one does not have control because few choices are available. This may include choices in terms of housing, employment, and educational opportunities, or even for the young black female, the choice of a young black male (considering the deaths due to homicide among this population).

Influence of Social Support and Family Interaction

Baekeland and Lundwall (1975), in an early review of the literature on patients dropping out of treatment, indicate that both social support and information about regimens positively predict patient adherence. For example, these authors found, in reviewing nineteen studies of social support and dropping out of treatment, that dropping out was associated with low social support in all of the studies. The studies covered a wide range of health problems, for example, alcoholism, hypertension, and emotional illness.

A selective review of the literature by Becker and Maiman (1975) looked at compliance with medical advice within the framework of patient-family interaction. Their findings suggest a complex set of relationships between health-related attitudes and motivations of family members and subsequent adoption of health behaviors by the patient. They state:

> The data suggests more attention be paid to the development of methods of educational interventions designed to modify relevant psychosocial variables in those individuals responsible for the health care of others in the family. (p. 176)

Also apparent in their review is that simple communications, role modeling, deliberate pressure, and family beliefs and behaviors positively affected family members' health actions. Similarly, the suggestion is that attitudes and behavioral patterns in the family often serve as barriers that interfere with compliance, especially when the family does not understand or support the regimen, or when family patterns are not consistent with requirements of the regimen.

Clearly, these findings have implications for African Americans as well as the population as a whole. These findings have implications for understanding many illnesses and problems in the black community, including those previously mentioned, that is, hypertension and infant mortality. It is not the intention here to go into the complex economic, historical, and social factors relating to the black family, which offers the primary social support. One must point out, however, that health professionals, policymakers, and others need to understand more about the black family and community and develop interventions and programs directly related to this understanding. Professionals need to understand that black churches, for example, offer a real support network for the black family and would often be more than willing to offer the use of the church for health meetings or support groups for both teens and adults. Policymakers interested in real prevention need to develop the leadership of the church and of the broader community into a political base strong and focused enough to empower the neighborhood (Kantor, 1990).

A CONCEPTUAL MODEL
TO INCREASE MEDICAL COMPLIANCE
AND PROMOTE HEALTH PREVENTION PROGRAMS

The results of these early studies with regard to influence of social support on compliance have continued to be confirmed over the years (Cramer and Spilker, 1991; Gerber and Nehemkis, 1986). Also, for example, the significance of social support in promoting compliance has been recently shown with hemodialysis patients (Boyer, Friend, and Chlouverkis, 1990) and with treating hypertensive patients (Dunbar, Dwyer, and Dunning, 1991). Thus, the significance of spousal or family support in promoting health compliance behavior is now quite recognized and must be given the utmost consideration in developing effective strategies or a working model to affect this problem.

Much of the current research related to health behavior and educational interventions has been based on the health belief model. The health belief model postulates that one's health behavior is influenced by one's belief according to

1. the extent to which individuals believe they are susceptible to disease;
2. how serious they think the disease would be should it occur, and the likelihood that the disease would occur without a change in behavior; and
3. how beneficial they believe certain actions would be in reducing their susceptibility to, or the severity of, the condition.

Green (Green et al., 1980) has developed a framework for health education built on the health belief model and on the basis of the cumulative research on health behavior. He identified three classes of factors that have potential for affecting behavior. These he classifies as *predisposing* factors, *enabling* factors, and *reinforcing* factors:

> *Predisposing* factors are a person's attitudes, beliefs, values, and perceptions that facilitate or hinder personal motivation for change. *Enabling* factors are considered to be barriers created mainly by societal forces or systems, e.g., limited facilities, inadequate personal or community resources, lack of income or health insurance, and even restrictive laws and statutes. The skills and knowledge required for a desired behavior to occur also qualify as enabling factors. *Reinforcing* factors are those factors related to the feedback the learner receives from others, either to encourage or to discourage behavioral change. (Green et al., 1980, p. 16)

To be most effective, then, interventions must occur that impact on each of these three classes of factors. The major health and patient education efforts today, largely occurring in the field of nursing, concentrate on merely increasing the patient's or family's knowledge of the illness or of the medical regimen. These efforts are largely directed at individual patients or groups of patients with specific diseases and frequently are concerned with providing information about diet, medications, and specific instructions, or, in other words, affecting a small part of the predisposing and the enabling factors. These are, of course, very important functions. However, this approach or focus may often be the reason these studies do not reveal that health education has a significant impact on adherence. Perhaps even worse is the observation that health care providers seldom behave according to research recommendations (Sluijs and Knibbe, 1991).

In addition, a basic contradiction exists in the idea of "compliance," "locus of control," and patient adult health education. Compliance implies a degree of control or authority that is often repugnant to many educators, as it suggests subservience, dependence, and unquestioning obedience to authority (Squires, 1980).

Many authorities today see compliance as being antithetical to the ideas of participatory concepts and believe it also fails to adequately consider the needs of the individual and the rights of self-determination and privacy (Bentley, Rosenson, and Zito, 1990; Trastie, 1989).

What is therefore needed are educational/behavioral-oriented strategies and interventions that incorporate the health belief model, the classes and factors outlined by Green, the basic principles of adult education with its participatory approach, and the concepts of problem solving and empowerment. This educational/behavioral intervention must emphasize consideration of the influences of the social system, family interaction, and social support reviewed in the previous section. Educational/behavioral interventions directed at problem-solving skills development occurring in a participatory climate (such as participatory self-help groups, for example) would relate to the enabling factors mentioned by Green. Compliance, therefore, must be considered in a multidimensional context or framework.

Bentley, Rosenson, and Zito (1990) have observed that problem-solving skills include defining problems, brainstorming solutions, discussing pros and cons, and choosing active strategies. Interventions in this area could be accomplished in a family, social, or community context, with the emphasis placed on the individual, family, or community to take responsibility for personal health behaviors. The black community has begun to take steps in this direction. It understands the need for self-help and leadership and is addressing the growing crisis among children and families. During the past decade, almost every major black organization has made preventing teen pregnancy and strengthening black families important priorities. These organizations, to name but a few, include the Children's Defense Fund, the National Council of Negro Women, the National Coalition of 100 Black Women, the Black Catholic Women of the Knights of Peter Claver, and the National Urban League (White, 1994).

Daphne Busby discusses the results of such organizing efforts in her essay "Single Mothers in Brooklyn." The network developed by the National Women's Health Project referred to in the essay has enabled and empowered the strengths of these women to organize and develop their leadership skills. Busby does, however, say that the lack of "total commitment of Black churches to become involved politically in health projects and concerns" is a considerable obstacle (Busby, 1990, p. 87).

Furthermore, patients need not only to become participants in their own health care decisions but also to be able to develop skills in gaining access to health care systems. This may include developing problem-solving skills, defining for themselves the questions to ask the physician regarding health matters, developing assertiveness necessary to participate in their own health decisions and care, and obtaining information they define as necessary for good health.

Efforts at developing or enhancing these skills in individuals, families, and communities result in the enhancement of self-worth and in the development of overall coping skills. Teaching decision-making skills may be as important as giving more instruction on taking medication. As may be seen, this would likely lead to the empowerment of the individual, family, and community, enabling them to begin taking responsibility for their health behaviors. Interventions should then also focus on the development of leaders and volunteers in the community who have influence and who may have the greatest impact upon the family. The black community has recently been working in this area (Cornelius, 1993).

SUMMARY AND CONCLUSION

The extensive review of the literature here leads to the conclusion that medical compliance cannot just be "taught"; individuals, families, and communities must become involved, committed, and responsible—in other words, empowered. They must become empowered to develop their own best system for following medical recommendations, to develop their own plans at community and family health prevention and promotion programs, and empowered to develop the necessary resources and access to resources to accomplish their goals (Sewell, 1995).

It may be that a new type of health care worker is needed, not only a health educator to pass out leaflets or a public health worker to determine from whom someone contracted a sexually transmitted disease, for example, but, rather, a preventive health care specialist or similar person trained in health education, public health, and the aspects of individual, family, and community systems intervention.

In other words, this new professional must, in many ways, be akin to the indigenous health care workers in China who know the individuals, families, and the communities in which they work. This new professional must be prepared to focus on all of the factors previously mentioned: the predisposing, enabling, and reinforcing components of the equation. This professional might assist individuals and lay volunteers in teaching problem-solving and coping skills, and in helping to create a climate in the family and in the community whereby these groups may feel empowered to inform the "elite" about how medical care is and is not working for them as individuals, and how illnesses and the medical system are affecting their community. High-risk populations have had little contact or voice in their own health care. This may be the only way toward compliance and prevention.

REFERENCES

Agras, W.S. (1989). Understanding compliance with the medical regimen: The scope of the problem and a theoretical perspective. *Arthritis Care and Research, 2*(1), 82-87.

Baekeland, F. and Lundwall, L. (1975). Dropping out of treatment. *Psychological Bulletin, 82*(4), 738-783.

Becker, M.H. and Maiman, L.A. (1975). Sociobehavioral determinants of compliance with health and medical recommendations. *Medical Care, 13*(1), 10-24.

Bentley, K.J., Rosenson, M.K., and Zito, J.M. (1990). Promoting medication compliance strategies for working with families of mentally ill people. *Social Work, 35*(2), 274-277.

Boyer, C.B., Friend, R., and Chlouverkis, G. (1990). Social support and demographic factors influencing compliance of hemodialysis patients. *Applied Social Psychology, 20*(4), 1902-1918.

Busby, D. (1990). Single mothers in Brooklyn. *Political Science Quarterly, 105*(1), 142.

Cohen, S.J. (Ed.) (1979). *New directions in patient compliance* (p. 1). Toronto: Lexington Books.

Cornelius, L. (1993). Health. In M.W. Williams and M. Cavendish (Eds.), *African American encyclopedia* (pp. 734-744). New York: Marshall Cavendish.

Cramer, J.A. and Spilker, B. (Eds.) (1991). *Patient compliance in medical practice and clinical trials.* New York: Raven Press.

Donovan, J.L. and Blake, D.R. (1992). Patient non-compliance: Deviance or reasoned decision-making. *Social Science and Medicine, 34*(3), 507-513.

Dunbar, J., Marshall, G., and Hovell, M. (1979). Behavioral strategies for improving compliance. In R.B. Haynes, D.W. Taylor, and D.L. Sackett (Eds.), *Compliance in health care* (pp. 174-190). Baltimore, MD: Johns Hopkins University Press.

Dunbar, J., Dwyer, K., and Dunning, J.E. (1991). Compliance with anti-hypertensive regimen: A review of the research in the 1980s. *Annals of Behavioral Medicine, 13*(1), 31-39.

Gerber, K.E. and Nehemkis, A.M. (Eds.) (1986), *Compliance: The dilemma of the chronically ill.* New York: Springer Publishing Company.

Green, L. (1979). Educational strategies to improve compliance and therapeutic and preventive regimens: The recent evidence. In R.B. Haynes, D.W. Taylor, and D.L. Sackett (Eds.), *Compliance in health care* (pp. 157-173). Baltimore, MD: Johns Hopkins University Press.

Green, L.W., Fisher, A., Amin, R., and Shafiullah, A.B.M. (1980). *Health education planning—A diagnostic approach.* Palo Alto, CA: Mayfield.

Greenburg, M. and Schneider, D. (1995). Health promotion priorities of economically stressed cities. *Journal of Health Care for the Poor and Disadvantaged, 6*(1), 10.

Haynes, R.B., Taylor, D.W., and Sackett, D. (Eds.) (1979). *Compliance in health care.* Baltimore, MD: Johns Hopkins University Press.

Kantor, P. (1990). The struggles for black empowerment in New York City: Beyond the politics of pigmentation (a book review). *The Political Science Quarterly, 105,* 162.

Levy, R. and Carter, R.L. (1976). Compliance with practitioner instigations. *Social Work, 4*(2), 188-193.

Marston, M. (1970). Compliance with medical regimens: A review of the literature. *Nursing Research, 19*(2), 312-322.

Morisky, D.E. (1990). A patient education program to improve adherence rates with anti-tuberculosis drug regimens. *Health Education Quarterly, 17*(2), 253-257.

Prothrow-Stith, D. (1995). The epidemic of youth violence in America: Using public health prevention strategies to prevent violence. *Journal of Health Care for the Poor and Underserved, 6*(1), 94.

Sewell, T. (1995). The pulling power of empowerment. *The Voice, 4*(3), 667.

Sluijs, E.M. and Knibbe, J.J. (1991). Patient compliance with exercises: Different theoretical approaches to short-term and long-term compliance. *Patient Education and Counseling, 17*(2), 191-204.

Squires, W.D. (Ed.) (1980). *Patient education.* New York: Springer Publishing Company.

Trastie, J.A. (1989). Medical compliance as an ideology. *Social Science and Medicine, 27*(5), 1299-1308.

Trick, L.R. (1993). Medical compliance—Patient compliance: Don't count on it. *Journal of the American Optometric Association, 64,* 264-270.

White, E.C. (1994). *The black women's health book.* Seattle, WA: Seal Press.

Zongas, T., Barr, C., and Barsky, A. (1991). Prediction of compliance with medication and follow-up appointments. *Nordisk Psykiatrisk Tideskrift, 45,* 27-32.

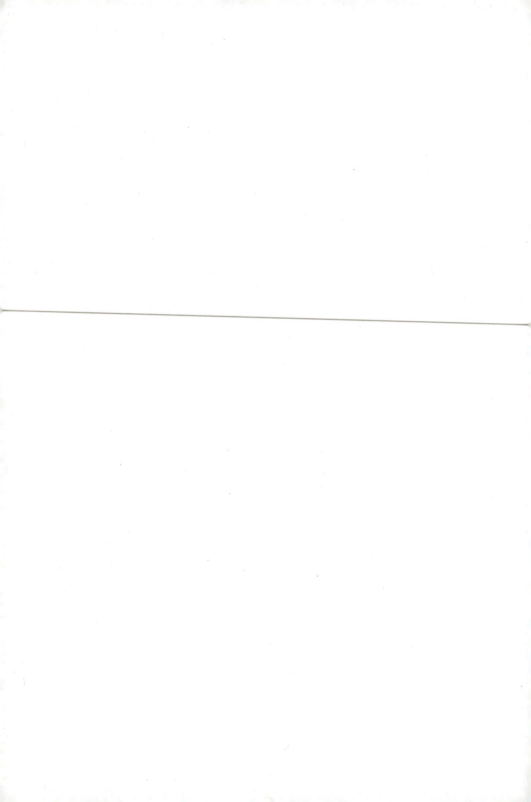

Chapter 6

The Impact of Infertility in the Black Community

Valerie Montgomery-Rice
Gloria Richard-Davis

INTRODUCTION

Infertility affects the black community at the same rate as the majority population in the United States. The currently accepted medical definition of infertility is one year of unprotected intercourse without conception. Based on this definition, 10 to 20 percent of married couples in the United States will experience infertility. Data collected by the National Center for Health Statistics estimates that in 1990, 2.3 million couples had impaired fertility (Jaffe and Jewelewicz, 1991). These data are not collected by ethnic groups. Therefore, the exact incidence of infertility in the black population is unknown. The reported information has been obtained from fertility centers, nationally and generally, that serve middle- to upper-socioeconomic-status patients. Currently, no database on infertility in blacks exists. However, some authors assume that infertility rates are lower in black communities. In addition, one misconception is that tubal disease resulting from sexually transmitted disease is a more common infertility factor in black patients. Therefore, the purpose of this chapter is threefold: to highlight this important area of study regarding the reproductive needs of African-American families; to emphasize the need for larger, more systematic studies on black infertility and its impact in the communities and on families; and to provide basic information regarding methods for understanding and responding to infertility.

EPIDEMIOLOGY

Several epidemiological factors contribute to infertility. Many couples are delaying childbearing, making age a major factor. The maximal reproductive capacity for women is between the ages of twenty-one and twenty-four and gradually declines thereafter (Moghissi, 1979a). This coincides with the time in which many women are also developing their careers and delaying their decision to have children. In addition, advancing age increases the risk of exposure to diseases such as endometriosis, sexually transmitted disease (STDs), and pelvic inflammatory disease (PID), all of which can potentially impair one's normal fertility and ability to achieve a pregnancy. Men are most fertile between the ages of twenty-four to twenty-five years. However, there have been reported cases of men fathering children well into their sixties (Moghissi, 1979b).

Several environmental effects have an impact on fertility: Nicotine and other components of cigarette smoke adversely affect cervical mucus, tubal motility, sperm development, and oocyte viability. Illicit drugs (marijuana, narcotics) can affect hormone secretion as well as impair sperm production and motility (Jaffe and Jewelewicz, 1991). Environmental and occupational exposures to ionizing radiation, textile dyes, and numerous other chemicals may have an adverse effect on female and male fertility as well (Speroff, Glass, and Kase, 1989).

Fertility is also related to the frequency of intercourse. Excessive coital activity may result in a decline in sperm density. However, for most men with normal counts, consecutive days of ejaculation will only decrease the count by 20 percent (Brown et al., 1997). Infrequent coitus reduces the chance of the sperm and egg encounter, thereby decreasing the chances of conception.

ETIOLOGY

In most studies, the causes of infertility are similar. In order of prevalence, causes include sperm defect (30 percent); ovulatory dysfunction (20 to 30 percent); tubal disease (15 to 30 percent); unexplained infertility (15 percent); cervical and uterine factors, including fibroids (10 percent); and endometriosis (4 to 6 percent) (Jaffe and Jewelewicz, 1991; Speroff, Glass, and Kase, 1989). Infertility may have multiple etiologies in many couples, all of which should be evaluated (see Figure 6.1).

The incidence of any individual factor can only be estimated and varies with the study population. In an attempt to determine the infertility factors that might specifically affect the black community, we surveyed new infertility patients presenting to an urban medical center, with greater than 90 percent of the couples surveyed being African American. All patients who attended our clinic between January 1, 1996, and April 15, 1997, were interviewed by either a medical student or a resident. Informed consent, as approved by an institutional review board, was obtained prior to the interview. The first of two pages of the questionnaire was completed at the initial visit. Questionnaires designed to obtain information on demographics, general health practices, and clinical information on factors affecting fertility were administered to new infertility patients by nurses and physicians. Information obtained included demographics such as age, race, length of infertility, and tobacco and alcohol use. A general gynecological history, detailing information about previous pregnancies, menstrual cycle, sexually transmitted diseases, previous contraceptive methods, and Pap smear, was obtained at that time. A sexual history was also elicited, and specific information on vaginal douching was obtained. A comprehensive physical exam was then performed, and the appropriate initial laboratory tests were ordered. The questionnaire was then filed in the chart. Infertility evaluation of the couple was obtained in a traditional manner, as outlined in Figures 6.1 and 6.2.

The demographics of the 103 couples in the final study group are shown in Table 6.1. The ages of the women ranged from 21 to 40, with a mean of 30.6 years, whereas the men ranged from 23 to 58 years, with a mean of 33.6 years. The average height of the women was 5 feet 5 inches, and the average weight was 204 pounds. The majority of the participants tended to be African American (>90 percent) and of lower socioeconomic status (SES). The lower SES was demonstrated by the level of education (12 percent had less than a high school education) and family income (approximately 90 percent of the couples reported a family income of less than

FIGURE 6.1. Basic Fertility Survey

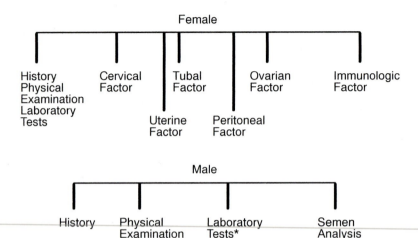

*Laboratory tests may include FSH, LH, TSH, P, hysterosalpingogram.

$15,000 per year). Only 23 percent of our patients reported smoking, and fewer than 10 percent reported alcohol consumption.

Secondary infertility was more common than primary infertility (64 percent versus 39 percent). Of the patients, 80 percent had had a Pap smear, with 75 percent within the last year; 80 percent reported douching. Of the women who reported douching, 40 percent, compared with 27 percent of those who did not, also reported a history of PID. This was not found to be statistically significant ($P = 1.0$). Of the patients, 40 percent reported a history of a pelvic infection, with chlamydia being the most frequently cited pathogen (>70 percent). Of those patients reporting a history of PID, 50 percent were diagnosed with tubal factor. This was statistically significant ($P < 0.0001$). The association of smoking with tubal factor was then examined (see Table 6.2). [Of smokers, 35 percent had tubal factor, compared to 25 percent of nonsmokers. This was not statistically significant ($P > 1.000$)]. In examining the variable of time to conception, most patients (>70 percent) attending the clinic had been attempting pregnancy for less than three years. Of patients who have been attempting pregnancy for more than five years, the factor most

FIGURE 6.2. Optimal Time for Various Infertility Investigations

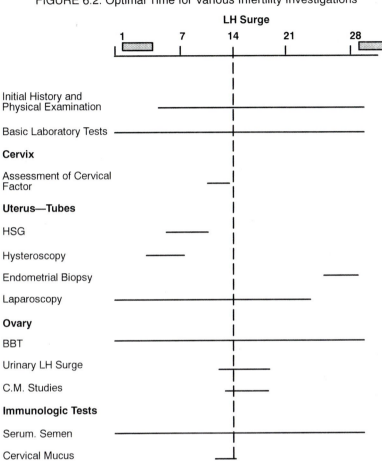

Note: HSG = hysterosalpingogram; BBT = basal body temperature.

commonly diagnosed was that of ovulatory dysfunction (>50 percent of the time), while in the less-than-three-years group, the most common factor was almost equally divided between the tubal and ovarian factors. The overall findings are as follows. Female infertility: when

TABLE 6.1. Demographic Characteristics of the Population

Average Age	30.6 years (women) 33.6 years (men)	
Ethnicity	African American	92.0%
	Caucasian	7.0%
	Others	< 1.0%
Education	Less than high school	12.0%
	High school	81.0%
	Greater than high school	7.0%
Family Income	Less than $15,000	89.0%
	Greater than $15,000	11.0%
Alcohol Consumption		9.8%
Tobacco Use		23.0%

TABLE 6.2. Tubal Factor in Patients Who Smoke or Douche

	Tubal Factor	**No Tubal Factor**
Smokers	35%	65%
Nonsmokers	25%	75%
Douching	40%	60%
Nondouching	27%	73%

only considering female factors, ovarian factors account for 42 percent (43 patients [pts]); tubal factor, 34 percent (35 pts); endometrial-uterine factor, 11 percent (12 pts); peritoneal factor, 6 percent (5 pts), and cervical factor (<1 percent). Only twenty-five males provided specimens for semen analysis; therefore, male factor could only be evaluated in these twenty-five patients. In that subset of twenty-five couples, infertility was thus reported as male factor, 29 percent; ovulatory, 38 percent; tubal, 39 percent.

The results suggest that infertility patients in an urban setting have the same distribution of causative factors as those in private, middle-class practices. Ovulatory dysfunction was the most common factor cited in both populations. This contradicts the belief that there is an increased prevalence of pelvic infection and subsequent increased tubal factor in low-income patients. In our study population, pelvic infection was historically reported in 40 percent of patients, and 50 percent of those patients have tubal factor. Therefore, the relationship between pelvic infection and tubal disease is significant. However, ovulatory dysfunction was still more prevalent. In our population, ovulatory dysfunction may also be linked to obesity. Studies have shown that obesity interferes with normal ovulation (Pratt et al., 1985). The average weight of women in our clinic was 204 pounds. Thus, even though tubal factor was common, ovulatory dysfunction was the most frequent factor.

Previous epidemiology reports of infertility noted that 30 percent of women reported smoking (Mueller and Daling, 1989), compared to our 23 percent. Cigarette smoking had previously been reported as a risk factor for pelvic infection and, thus, infertility (Baird and Wilcox, 1985; Howe et al., 1985; Phillips et al., 1992; Phipps et al., 1987; Scholes, Daling, and Stergachis, 1992; Stillman, Rosenberg, and Sachs, 1986). In our population, a higher percentage of the smokers had PID compared to the nonsmokers (35 percent versus 25 percent). Several studies reported an association between douching and pelvic inflammatory disease, as well as pelvic inflammatory disease and subsequent tubal pregnancy (Aral, Mosher, and Cates, 1988; Baird et al., 1996; Chow et al., 1985; Daling et al., 1991; Forrest et al., 1989; Scholes et al., 1993). In a nationally representative sample of 8,459 U.S. females between the ages of fifteen and forty-four, it was noted that 37 percent of patients douche (Aral, Mosher, and Cates, 1988), in comparison to 80 percent in our study population. It was reported that the variable most strongly and consistently associated with douching was race: two-thirds of black women, but only one-third of white women douche. It was also noted more frequently among thirty- to thirty-four-year-old women who lived in poverty and those with less than a high school education. This is consistent with the demographics of our population (see Table 6.1), a lower socioeconomic status and predominantly African American. In their population (Aral, Mosher, and Cates, 1988), 16 percent of women who reported douching also reported a history of PID. Our study showed a higher frequency of tubal factors among women who douched; however, it was not statistically significant. Women in the thirty to forty age group who douched had a higher frequency of tubal pregnancy compared to the twenty to thirty age group. Since douching has been shown to be a modifiable risk factor for PID and possible tubal pregnancy, extensive education is needed to decrease this practice in the black community.

The final variable examined was time to conception. In our patient population, ovulatory dysfunction was the most common factor noted in patients attempting pregnancy for more than five years. This time factor may be attributable to limited continued treatment options (such as in vitro fertilization) in lower SES patients with tubal factor, suggesting that patients with tubal factor treated surgically either conceive within two years or discontinue treatment in our facility.

EVALUATION

Based on the findings from our survey, infertility factors affecting African-American couples are identical to those reported in the literature. Therefore, evaluation and treatment of those couples should follow the standard approach. A thorough evaluation would include the following components.

History

Every effort should be made to initiate the fertility evaluation with a joint interview of the couple that includes a comprehensive medical and surgical history of both partners. The woman should be questioned regarding menstrual cycle, pregnancy, contraceptive use, and sexual history. Details relating to coital frequency and timing, sexual dysfunction, and possible use of lubricants should be obtained. The man should be questioned about his fertility and sexual history. A social history and record of exposure to environmental and occupational toxins should be elicited from both partners. Finally, any prior workup or treatment for infertility should be noted, and all pertinent records should be obtained. Suggested time guidelines for infertility investigations are found in Figure 6.2.

Physical Examination

The general examination should be comprehensive, as the gynecologist is often the woman's primary care physician. Special attention should be directed at height, weight, presence of galactorrhea or acne, breast size, and hair distribution. The pelvic examination should screen for any anatomic or pathologic abnormalities (e.g., masses, infection, endometriosis). Examination of the man should include evaluation of the external genitalia, size and consistency of the testicles, presence of congenital anomalies (e.g., undescended testicles), and varicocele.

Laboratory Evaluation

Preliminary laboratory tests should include urinalysis, complete blood cell count, rubella titer, and a serologic syphilis test for both partners. Additional tests for the woman may include thyroid stimulating hormone (TSH), serum prolactin (P), follicle-stimulating hormone (FSH), luteinizing hormone (LH), testosterone, dehydroepiandrosterone sulfate (DHEAS), 17-hydroxyprogesterone, and chromosomal studies, as indicated.

FEMALE FACTORS

Ovulation

Ovulation disorders account for approximately 20 percent of all infertility (Speroff, Glass, and Kase, 1989). Ovulation usually occurs in most women who menstruate regularly. However, even in women who exhibit cyclic bleeding, occasional anovulatory cycles may occur. A more important (and frequently unrecognized) disturbance of the ovulatory process is the presence of luteal-phase defects (LPD) or an inadequate or short luteal phase.

Ovulation is evaluated indirectly via basal body temperature (BBT), steroid or gonadotropin hormone assays, ultrasonography, cervical mucus changes, or endometrial biopsy. Ovulation should be evaluated for several cycles. BBT is the oldest, most widely used method of ovulation detection. A sharp rise of 0.4 to 0.6°C between two consecutive days generally indicates ovulation. Ovulation has been reported to occur in 3 to 20 percent of monophasic BBTs and may be absent in a small percentage of biphasic BBTs (Barad, 1991).

The midcycle serum LH surge is the most reliable predictor of ovulation but is expensive to analyze and requires frequent blood sampling. Urinary LH kits are now available commercially and are a reasonable alternative; the evening radioimmunoassay (RIA) urine LH kit was found to detect the day of surge correctly in 98 percent of women (Jaffe and Jewelewicz, 1991).

Endometrial biopsy can both confirm ovulation and evaluate the adequacy of the luteal phase. Although diagnosis and treatment of LPD remains controversial, it is generally accepted that the diagnosis requires two endometrial biopsies to be two or more days out of phase. The luteal phase is inadequate in up to 30 percent of cycles in normal women (Jaffe and Jewelewicz, 1991). The incidence of recurrent LPD in the infertile population ranges from 3 to 14 percent (Jaffe and Jewelewicz, 1991).

Cervical Factors

A cervical factor accounts for approximately 5 to 10 percent of infertility (Moghissi, 1979b). Although the postcoital test (PCT)—also known as the Simms-Huhner test—is accepted as an integral part of the infertility workup, its interpretation is controversial. Gross and microscopic examination of the cervical mucus should be performed at, or immediately before, the time of ovulation. The motility of spermatozoa and the cervical mucus grade have been classified by Moghissi (1979b) (see Figure 6.3). Grossly, the quantity (0 to more than 0.3 milliliter [ml]), viscosity (viscous to watery), and stretchability, or spinnbarkheit (0 to more than 8 centimeters [cm]), is assessed and assigned a score of 0 to 3.

Microscopically, the fern pattern (simple to tertiary branching), cellularity per high-power field (HPF) (many to fewer than 5), and motile sperm per HPF (immotile to vigorous forward motility) are observed and scored 0 to 3. Under ideal conditions, more than 10 sperm per HPF with grades 3+ motility constitutes a normal result.

The optimal interval after intercourse to obtain a PCT is debatable; recommendations vary from 2 to 24 hours (h). Since complement-dependent reactions that immobilize sperm require 8 to 10 h to occur, an 8 to 12 h interval may be best (Bronson, Cooper, and Rosenfeld, 1984). Abnormal PCT findings may result from inappropriate timing, inadequate estrogen levels, vaginal or cervical

FIGURE 6.3. Cervical Score (A Composite of the Amount, Spinnbarkheit, Ferning, Viscosity, and Cellularity of Cervical Mucus)

Amount	None	0
	0.1 ml	1
	0.2 ml	2
	0.3 ml or greater	3
Spinnbarkheit	None	0
	1-4 cm	1
	5-8 cm	2
	9 cm or greater	3
Ferning	None	0
	Atypical (1+)	1
	2+	2
	3 or 4+	3
Viscosity	4+	0
	3+	1
	2+	2
	1+	3
Cellularity (HPF × 400)	11 or greater	0
	8-10	1
	1-5	2
	Occasional	3

Note: Maximum score is 15; scores less than 10 represent unfavorable mucus, and scores less than 5 represent hostile cervical secretion.

infection, inadequate cervical mucus production, or the presence of sperm antibodies.

Tubal/Uterine Factors

Although tubal factors may be responsible for 20 percent of infertility, uterine abnormalities are a factor in only about 2 percent (Hammond and Talbert, 1985). The common uterine abnormality seen is leiomyomata or fibroids. The current procedure for initial evaluation of uterine and tubal factors is hysterosalpingography (HSG), which has a correlation of about 75 percent with laparoscopy or hysteroscopy for accuracy (Hammond and Talbert, 1985). The procedure should be performed in the early follicular phase after menses has stopped and should be postponed if there is any evidence of infection or a pelvic mass. The risk of an infection from the procedure is less than 1 percent in low-risk populations and 3 percent in high-risk populations (e.g., those with a history of pelvic inflammatory disease, septic abortion, intrauterine device [IUD] usage, ruptured appendix, pelvic or tubal surgery, or ectopic pregnancy). The therapeutic effects of HSG remain controversial. If the findings are normal, six months should be allowed for the appearance of possible therapeutic benefits before initiating operative procedures.

Hysteroscopy and laparoscopy are the final diagnostic procedures of the basic infertility workup. Hysteroscopy is best scheduled after menses and before ovulation. It should be performed by an experienced gynecologist who can proceed with surgery, if indicated. When used as a diagnostic procedure of last resort, laparoscopy has a high incidence of detecting endometriosis and pelvic adhesions. Therefore, laser or operative laparoscopy should be readily available.

Congenital anomalies, uterine fibroids, and polyps may cause uterine cavity distortion. Uterine fibroids, however, are the most common cause of uterine distortion. The incidence of fibroids in the general population is 20 to 40 percent. However, fibroids are three to four times more common in African-American women than among white women (Marshalal et al., 1977). The exact cause of fibroids is unknown. Fibroids may be located in the submucosal, intramural, or subserosal area. Subserosal fibroids have generally been accepted to decrease fertility by impeding implantation in the endometrial cavity. Recent studies, however, have revealed a decrease in fertility in patients with fibroids located intramurally, as well as submucosally (Elder-Geva et al., 1997; Farhi et al., 1995). Therefore, fibroids should definitely be removed if distortion of the endometrial cavity is documented by HSG or hysteroscopy. In addition, consideration should be given to removing any intramural fibroids greater than 3 cm in infertile women (Elder-Geva et al., 1997).

MALE FACTORS

Semen samples should be obtained for analysis by masturbation into a clean container after two to three days of abstinence from intercourse. The sample is best produced in an area adjacent to the laboratory but may also be obtained at home, kept warm, and delivered to a reliable laboratory within 1 h. Two or three semen analyses at two-week intervals are necessary to provide a reasonable assessment of male fertility.

Even with sophisticated techniques, semen analysis provides only a rough measure of the functional ability of sperm. The basic semen analysis assesses the physical characteristics of the semen and the sperm density, motility, and morphology. World Health Organization (WHO) criteria for normal values of semen variables are shown in Table 6.3 (WHO, 1992). The exact parameters for normal results are difficult to determine. Numerous studies have shown that couples can conceive with abnormal semen findings, suggesting that sperm motility and morphology correlate better with pregnancy than sperm density (Dunphy, Neal, and Cooke, 1989). Factors resulting in abnormal semen findings may include stress; infection; certain medications; use of tobacco, alcohol, or illicit drugs; tight underwear; or frequent hot baths.

TABLE 6.3. Standard Semen Analysis

Volume	≥ 2.0 ml
pH	7.2-8.0
Sperm concentration	$\geq 20 \times 10^6$ spermatozoa per ml
Total sperm count	$\geq 40 \times 10^6$ spermatozoa per ejaculate
Motility	$\geq 50\%$ with forward progression (categories a and b) or $\geq 25\%$ with rapid progression (category a) within 60 min of ejaculation
Morphology	$\geq 30\%$ with normal forms
Vitality	$\geq 75\%$ live (i.e., excluding dye)
White blood cells	$<1 \times 10^6$ per ml
Immunobased test	<20% spermatozoa with adherent particles
Mix antiglobulin reaction (MAR) test	<10% spermatozoa with adherent particles

Source: Adapted from WHO, 1992.

In some cases, there is still a question of male-factor infertility despite normal semen findings. If a complete evaluation of the woman reveals no abnormality, further studies, such as the sperm penetration assay (SPA) or computer-assisted sperm movement analysis (CASMA), should be performed to evaluate sperm function. The SPA evaluates the interaction of sperm with a hamster egg after the removal of the zona pellucida, measuring capacitation, acrosome reaction, membrane fusion, incorporation into the ooplasm, and decondensation of the sperm chromatin. SPA results are reported as the number of sperm penetrating per ovum; a mean of 5 is considered to be the lower limits of normal. With the exception of zona penetration, this test mimics in vitro fertilization.

CASMA allows detailed analysis of the motion characteristics of individual sperm—e.g., velocity, linearity, lateral head displacement—that may be important in determining fertilization capacity. Several studies have documented differences in movement patterns between sperm of fertile and infertile men (Ginsburg, 1993). The relationship between movement and the capacity to fertilize is unclear at present.

OTHER FACTORS

Studies have reported a greater prevalence of genital mycoplasma in the cervical mucus and semen of infertile couples than of fertile couples (Cassel et al., 1983; Fowlkes, MacLeod, and O'Leary, 1975; Friberg, 1980; Speroff, Glass, and Kase, 1994). Types recovered from the genital tract include *Mycoplasma hominis* and *Ureaplasma urealyticum*. Although the correlation between genital mycoplasma and infertility remains debatable, cultures should be obtained, and patients with positive findings should be treated with doxycycline. Antibodies to cervical mucus, sperm, and blood should be obtained if the PCT result is abnormal or in the case of sperm agglutination or unexplained infertility.

CONCLUSION

Ten to twenty percent of couples will experience infertility. Tubal and ovulatory factors are the major causes of infertility in the black community, which is not significantly different from the majority community. In our small subset of couples, male factor was lower than expected; however, this could be attributed to the small sample size. To fully understand the impact of infertility in the black community, larger observational studies are needed.

Although very few couples with infertility have a physical disability, their mental anguish may severely undermine their physical well-being, marital fulfillment, and family life. A well-informed and sympathetic physician who is capable of establishing a good rapport and initiating an orderly, meticulous, and comprehensive program of investigation and management can provide couples with an immense measure of comfort. With careful study, the etiology of infertility can be identified in almost 90 percent of couples. Pregnancies will occur in 40 to 50 percent of adequately evaluated and treated infertile couples. Sophisticated, innovative therapeutic modalities such as ovulation induction, microsurgery, and assisted reproductive technologies should further improve these results.

REFERENCES

Aral, S.O., Mosher, W.D., and Cates, W., Jr. (1988). Vaginal douching among women of reproductive age in the United States. *American Journal of Public Health, 82*(2), 210-214.

Baird, D.D., Weinberg, C.R., Voigt, L.F., and Daling, J.R. (1996). Vaginal douching and reduced fertility. *American Journal of Public Health, 86*(6), 844-850.

Baird, D.D. and Wilcox, A.J. (1985). Cigarette smoking associated with delayed conception. *Journal of the American Medical Association, 253*(10), 2979.

Barad, D. (1991). Workup of the infertile couple. In D. Barad (Ed.), *Infertility and reproductive medicine clinics of North America* (pp. 255-267). Philadelphia: W.B. Saunders.

Bronson, R.A., Cooper, G.W., and Rosenfeld, D.L. (1984). Autoimmunity to spermatozoa effect in sperm penetration of cervical mucus as reflected by postcoital testing. *Fertility Sterility, 14*(2), 609.

Brown, S.E., Montgomery-Rice, V.C., Stewart, D.L., Harris, M.A, Jordan, S., and Clinton, P.K. (1997). *Effects of consecutive ejaculation in the total number of mobile sperm inseminated* (Abstract #0-0090). The 53rd Annual Meeting of the American Society of Reproductive Medicine. Washington, DC: American Society of Reproductive Medicine.

Cassel, G.H., Younger, J.B., Brown, M.B., Blackwell, R., Davis, J.K., Marriott, P., and Stagno, S. (1983). Microbiologic study of infertile women at the time of diagnostic laparoscopy—Association of *Ureaplasma urealyticum* with a defined subpopulation. *New England Journal of Medicine, 308*(4), 502.

Chow, W.H., Daling, J.R., Weiss, N.S., Moore, D.E., and Soderstrom, R. (1985). Vaginal douching as a potential risk factor for tubal ectopic pregnancy. *American Journal of Obstetrics and Gynecology, 153*(7), 727-729.

Daling, J.R., Weiss, N.S., Schwartz, S.M., Stergachis, A., Wang, S.P., Foy, H., Chu, J., McKnight, B., and Grayston, J. (1991). Vaginal douching and the risk of tubal pregnancy. *Epidemiology, 2*(1), 40-48.

Dunphy, B.C., Neal, L.M., and Cooke, I.D. (1989). The clinical value of conventional semen analysis. *Fertility Sterility, 51*(3), 324.

Elder-Geva, T., Meagher, S., Healy, D.L., MacLachlan, V., Breheny, S., and Wood, C. (1997). Effects of intramural, subserosal and submucosal uterine fibroids on the outcome of assisted reproductive technology treatment. *Fertility Sterility, 70*(4), 687-691.

Farhi, J., Ashkenazi, J., Feldberg, D., Dicker, D.F.D., Orvieto, R., and Benrafael, Z. (1995). Effect of uterine leiomyomata on the results of in vitro fertilization treatment. *Human Reproduction, 10*(10), 2576-2578.

Forrest, K.A., Washington, A.E., Daling, J.R., and Sweet, R.L. (1989). Vaginal douching as a possible risk factor for pelvic inflammatory disease. *Journal of the National Medical Association, 81*(2), 159-165.

Fowlkes, D.M., MacLeod, J., and O'Leary, W.M. (1975). T-mycoplasmas and human infertility: Correlation of infection with alterations in seminal parameters. *Fertility Sterility, 26,* 1212.

Friberg, J. (1980). Mycoplasmas and ureaplasmas in infertility and abortion. *Fertility Sterility, 33,* 351.

Ginsburg, K. (1993). Computer-assisted sperm movement analysis. In W.D. Schlaff and J.A. Rock (Eds.), *Decision making in reproductive endocrinology* (pp. 438-443). Boston: Blackwell Scientific Publication.

Hammond, M.G. and Talbert, L.M. (1985). *Infertility: A practical guide for the physician* (Second edition). Oradell, NJ: Medical Economics Books.

Howe, G., Westhoff, C. Vessey, M., and Yeates, D. (1985). Effects of age, cigarette smoking and other factors in fertility: Findings in a large prospective study. *British Medical Journal, 290,* 1697.

Jaffe, S. and Jewelewicz, R. (1991). The basic infertility investigation. *Fertility Sterility, 56*(3), 599-613.

Marshalal, L.M., Speigelman, D., Barbieri, R.L., Goldman, M.B., Manson, J.E., Colditz, G.A., Willett, W.C., and Hunter, D.J. (1977). Variation in the incidence of uterine leiomyoma among premenopausal women by age and race. *Obstetrics and Gynecology, 90*(6), 967-973.

Moghissi, K. (1979a). Basic work-up and evaluation of infertile couples. In J.W. Pearson and K.M. Moghissi (Eds.), *Clinical obstetrics and gynecology* (pp. 11-25). Hagerstown, MD: Harper & Row.

Moghissi, K. (1979b). The cervix in infertility. In J.W. Pearson and K.M. Moghissi (Eds.), *Clinical obstetrics and gynecology* (pp. 27-37). Hagerstown, MD: Harper & Row.

Mueller, B.A., and Daling, J.R. (1989). Epidemiology of infertility. In M.R. Soules (Ed.), *Controversies in reproductive endocrinology and infertility* (p. 1). New York: Elsevier.

Phillips, R.S., Tuomala, R.E., Feldblum, P.J., Schachter, J., Rosenberg, M.J., and Aronson, M.D. (1992). The effect of cigarette smoking, *Chlamydia trachomatis* infection, and vaginal douching on ectopic pregnancy. *Obstetrics and Gynecology, 79*(1), 85-90.

Phipps, W.R., Cramer, D.W., Schiff, I., Belisle, S., Stillman, R., Albrecht, B., Gibson, M., Berger, M.J., and Wilson, E. (1987). The association between smoking and female infertility as influenced by cause of the fertility. *Fertility Sterility, 48*(2), 377.

Pratt, W.F., Mosher, W.D., Bachrach, C., and Horn, M.C. (1985). Infertility—United States, 1982. *Morbidity and Mortality Weekly Report, 34*(1), 197.

Scholes, D., Daling, J.R., and Stergachis, A.S. (1992). Current cigarette smoking and risk of acute pelvic inflammatory disease. *American Journal of Public Health, 82*(10), 1352-1355.

Scholes, D., Daling, J.R., Stergachis, A., Weiss, N.S., Wang, S.P., and Grayston, J.T. (1993). Vaginal douching as a risk factor for acute pelvic inflammatory disease. *Obstetrics and Gynecology, 81*(4), 601-606.

Speroff, L., Glass, R.H., and Kase, N.G. (1989). *Clinical gynecologic endocrinology and infertility* (Fourth edition) (pp. 513-546). Baltimore, MD: Williams and Wilkins.

Speroff, L., Glass, R.H., and Kase, N.G. (1994). *Clinical gynecologic endocrinology and infertility* (Fifth edition) Baltimore, MD: Williams and Wilkins.

Stillman, R.J., Rosenberg, M.J., and Sachs, B.P. (1986). Smoking and reproduction. *Fertility Sterility, 46*(1), 545.

World Health Organization (1992). *WHO laboratory manual for the examination of semen and semen-cervical mucus interaction* (Third edition) (p. 44). Cambridge: Cambridge University Press.

Chapter 7

The Health Care Needs of the Black Elderly: From Well to Frail

Brenda F. McGadney-Douglass

INTRODUCTION

Social workers are serving more elderly clients than ever before. Living longer, the American elderly population is growing at an alarming rate. In fact, the elderly population is expected to increase to 21.8 percent of the entire U.S. population by the year 2030 (Angel and Hogan, 1994). During the years 2020 and 2050, the most dramatic changes are projected to occur in the percentage among the oldest old (85+). Today's minorities constitute 14 percent of the older population; however, projections are that they will make up over one-third of those age sixty-five and older by the year 2050. Black American elders form the fastest growing segment of the black population, living in both rural and urban settings (Wykle and Kaskel, 1994).

The significance in the growth of the elderly population, particularly black Americans, to social workers employed in the health care field is that they must provide services to a very diverse population (e.g., beliefs, culture, ethnicity, socioeconomic status, disabilities and functional status, coping styles, language, health care practices and needs). It consists of elders who have physical and functional limitations associated with the aging process and others who are mentally retarded. Increasingly, elders with multiple chronic diseases and health problems are faced with disabilities and dependence due to a lack of preventive health care. About 70 percent of all deaths and a substantial amount of morbidity and disability in the United States are attributed to conditions such as heart disease, cancer, stroke, diabetes, chronic obstructive pulmonary disease (COPD), and cirrhosis. To address the impact of multiple chronic health problems among elders, social workers will be expected to promote wellness and health for them and their families by helping them to live independently in the community as long as possible. Thus, practitioners will want to help older persons, particularly black American elders, maintain the highest quality of life by facilitating effective service delivery based on their health care needs, beliefs, and practices.

Davis and Maryland (1997) provide a strong rationale for practitioners to promote wellness and health among elders:

> The graying of society coupled with the epidemiological transition (shift from infectious diseases to chronic diseases as leading causes of death) has stimulated greater interest in health promotion. Although effectiveness of health promotion has been documented, researchers and clinicians have given little attention to health promotion and the elderly. However, with more people living into the ninth and tenth decade of life, there has been a new focus on the elderly as noted in national reports, *Healthy People 2000* (U.S. Public Health Service, 1991) and forums such as the 1995 White House Mini Conference on Aging. (p. 97)

Given this background, the public health community has established a national health initiative known as *Healthy People 2000* (Public Health Service, 1991a). The Public Health Service has set a number of objectives for special populations that will reduce disparities in risk factors associated with morbidity and mortality from chronic diseases for elders, particularly black Americans (Truman et al., 1994; Public Health Service, 1991b, 1993). Social workers have a major role in empowering elders, families, and professional caregivers to meet these objectives in a collective endeavor to reduce the inequality in health among racial and ethnic groups, increase the span of healthy life for Americans, and provide access to preventive services for all Americans, particularly black American elders (Public Health Service, 1991a).

A variety of culturally sensitive preventive strategies exist that can be useful in promoting wellness among African-American elders (Cochran and McGadney, 1997; Davis, McGadney, and Perri, 1990a, b, c). Historically, blacks have engaged in self-care practices that have included various home remedies.

Black American elders engage in preventive self-care practices for a variety of reasons: (1) fragmentation of the health care system, (2) the use of lay consultation, (3) beliefs about the efficacy of treatment, and (4) perceived cause of illness (see Davis and McGadney, 1993, for more details). Therefore, to be effective, preventive practices for black Americans have to be influenced by a strong knowledge base of their cultural beliefs about chronic disease, illness, treatment (traditional and nontraditional), and wellness. To understand these beliefs, Cochran and McGadney (1997) suggest that practitioners must include in their assessments health beliefs (knowledge and compliance), behaviors (exercise and nutrition), and their service use among older black Americans.

To enhance social work knowledge of black American elders experiencing a range of health care needs, this chapter will include a discussion of the following components: (1) profile of chronic diseases, including leading causes of death and disabilities, and modifiable risk factors; (2) importance and role of collectivism in promoting health and wellness among elders; and (3) overview of three preventive interventions (primary, secondary, and tertiary), social work skills, and barriers to providing effective services.

CHRONIC HEALTH PROFILE
OF BLACK AMERICAN ELDERS

Heart disease, stroke, and cancer (lung, breast, and colorectal) are the leading causes of death for black Americans and for whites forty-five years or older. Available data on mortality and morbidity rates point out a number of striking differences and some commonalties between black Americans and whites. In 1990, black Americans had higher age-adjusted mortality rates for the same leading causes as did whites. For example, the death rate from diabetes for black American women is twice the rate for white women of comparable age, while black American men have lower mortality rates for ischemic heart disease (IHD), chronic obstructive pulmonary disease (COPD), and cirrhosis than do white men. However, black American men age sixty-five and older have a two times higher rate of prostate cancer than do white men. The leading causes of death among older black American men are IHD and lung cancer (followed by stroke); the two leading causes of death among black American women are IHD and stroke (followed by breast cancer).

These findings remain constant even after controlling for the different age structures of the two populations. They suggest commonalties in exposure to the causes of these diseases but differences between the groups in their exposures to determinants of death. Increased prevalence of smoking, hypertension, and obesity among black Americans are undoubtedly some of the causes for these higher mortality rates. Socioeconomic factors, such as poor living conditions (e.g., diet, sanitation, stress) and lack of access to quality health care, are more likely to influence disparities in mortality rates among black Americans than known biological risk factors (Otten et al., 1990; Pappas et al., 1993; Potter, 1991; Rogers, 1992; Sorlie et al., 1992).

Some data suggest that minority populations age biologically differently than whites. For example, relative to life expectancy, the "crossover phenomenon" shows that, proportionately, the hardiest of black Americans are more likely to outlive white Americans older than seventy-five. Researchers suggest that this crossover in life expectancy at age seventy-five results from selection and adaptation factors that cause surviving black American elders to be more hardy (American Association of Retired Persons, 1990b; Baker, 1988; O'Brien et al., 1989; Polednak, 1989). In 1990, black American life expectancy at birth was 9.1 years longer for females than for males (73.6 years versus 64.5 years) (National Center for Health Statistics, 1992). The survival advantage among black American females born in 1990 continued a trend of increasing life expectancies for black American males and females (Beckles, Blount, and Jiles, 1994). However, at all ages, life expectancies are higher for white adults than for black American adults.

Black American elders compared to whites, over the age of seventy-five, have lower mortality rates but have higher rates of poverty and morbidity. Findings from the National Health Interview Surveys, conducted from 1986-1990, show that black American elders reported the same leading chronic conditions as did whites but at generally higher levels. In descending order of prevalence, the conditions most commonly reported by black Americans were hypertension, diabetes, and cancer (Beckles, Blount, and Jiles, 1994).

The prevalence of self-reported hypertension was higher for black Americans than for whites for both sexes. Hypertension reached as high as 36.7 percent and 59.2 percent for sixty-five- to seventy-four-year-old men and women, respectively, then decreased to 30.3 percent and 54.8 percent among men and women ages seventy-five years and older.

Increasing with age, the prevalence for diabetes was 12.7 percent for men age sixty-five to seventy-four, and 14.2 percent for those seventy-five years and older; diabetes prevalence was 18.3 percent for women age sixty-five to seventy-four years, and 21.2 percent for those seventy-five years and older. Black American women had age-adjusted prevalences that were 80 percent higher for hypertension, 200 percent higher for diabetes, and 22 percent higher for stroke than those for white women. The age-adjusted prevalences for black American men were 34 percent higher for hypertension, 69 percent higher for diabetes, and 35 percent higher for stroke than the prevalences for white men.

Black Americans have the highest cancer incidence of any race/ethnic group in the United States (Clayton and Byrd, 1993; Miller et al., 1990). Regardless of race, the principal sites of cancer are the same, with the most common among black Americans being prostate for men, breast cancer for women, and lung and colorectal cancers for both sexes. Cancer of the breast is the most common cancer among black American women. Cancer of the lung and bronchus is the second most common cancer among black American men and the third most common among black American women. Colorectal cancer is the third most common cancer among black American men and the second most common among black American women.

Relative survival rates provide a measure of the effectiveness of medical intervention—early detection, access to clinical care, and the efficacy of care—on mortality caused by a specific cancer. Between 1983 and 1989, the five-year relative survival rates for black Americans were lower than those for whites for all cancer sites combined: 39 percent for black Americans and 55 percent for whites, except for the lung and stomach. The poorer survival rates found among black Americans for breast, cervical, and colorectal cancers suggest that factors such as low-quality health care, inadequate continuity of care, and insufficient access to optimal methods of detection, diagnosis, and treatment may be common among persons in this population (Miller et al., 1990).

Risk Factors and Preventive Health Behaviors

One comparative study by the Behavioral Risk Factor Surveillance System (BRFSS) identified in 1991 and 1992 the prevalence of selected risk factors and preventive health behaviors (e.g., sedentary lifestyle, obesity, smoking, high blood pressure, and cholesterol levels) among black American and white adults (Centers for Disease Control [CDC], 1992). Findings indicate that black Americans were more likely than whites to report a sedentary lifestyle in the previous month. More than three-quarters of black American adults who were sixty-five and older reported a sedentary lifestyle in the previous month. Black American adults were more likely to report that they were overweight than were white adults. The prevalence of self-reported overweight was highest for women ages forty-five to sixty-four (51.5 percent), with half being overweight.

Black Americans who were current smokers (one in five) were more likely than whites to report quitting for at least one day (CDC, 1992). The prevalence of persons who reported that they had their blood pressure checked was greater than 90 percent for black American adults and for white adults. In contrast, black Americans were less likely than whites to have their cholesterol levels checked. In all strata, black American women were more likely to report having had a recent Pap smear. However, the prevalence was lowest among women sixty-five and older, those with less than twelve years of education, and those who reported household incomes under $10,000. Among women fifty years and older, black Americans were less likely than whites to report that they had been screened for breast cancer within the two years before the interview. However, the prevalence of breast cancer was highest among black American elders.

COLLECTIVISM
AND BLACK HEALTH CARE PRACTICES

Current health promotion strategies focus primarily on empowering individual lifestyle practices—modification of risk at the individual level—particularly among well elders. Education, knowledge, and the development of skills are necessary to change behavior, but they are not sufficient. Social work agencies should collaborate with other agencies to develop and implement prevention strategies aimed at altering the social and physical environment to one that provides reinforcement for positive health choices at all levels of social work practice (and across the life span). Clinicians should seek to empower elders, families and friends, and formal care providers to work collectively to ensure quality health care for all elders in the community and those who are institutionalized.

Although some of the literature portrays a bleak image for the majority of minority elders, the accumulating evidence suggests that black American elders appear to rely on supportive relations with their children to resolve both their physical and psychological problems (McGadney and Madison, 1997; Taylor, 1985; Wykle and Kaskel, 1994).

It is well known that many African-American elderly enjoy extensive informal networks of family, friends, and church (Dilworth-Anderson, 1992; McGadney, 1992, 1995; Taylor, 1985). Socioeconomic and family factors (e.g., marital status, siblings in network) are known to influence these exchanges. Several issues are unique to African Americans compared to other American minority groups. They comprise the largest minority group in the United States, have one of the longest histories, and are the only group to have been relocated in this country involuntarily. The practice of black American elders to maintain good health is influenced by their cultural beliefs and behaviors, which are rooted in African traditions and blended with Southern traditions.

OVERVIEW OF INTERVENTIONS WITH THE ELDERLY

Social workers, as well as many others in the helping professions, will be asked to meet the challenges of providing services to a heterogeneous group of black American elders, ranging from the very healthy to the severely impaired. According to Zarit (1980), due to their unique experiences and lifestyle patterns, elders differ more widely from one another than do their younger cohorts. In fact, armed with a wealth of experiences, varying health conditions, and differing attitudes, behaviors, and levels of functional impairment associated with aging, elderly clients are possibly the most diverse group of clients with whom social workers will practice (Kropf and Hutchison, 1992). Therefore, based on their diverse backgrounds and abilities, interventions needed by the well elderly are different from those needed by the frail elderly. For example, need-based assistance for healthy elders may range from emphasizing well-balanced meals, exercise, and regular checkups to screenings for breast or prostate cancer and compliance with drug prescriptions. To address these differential needs, Beaver and Miller (1992) proposed three levels of interventions—primary, secondary, and tertiary—for effective social work practice with black American elders. A preventive approach is the most effective way to improve the quality of life for black elders and their families over a longer period of time.

Primary Prevention

"Primary prevention is viewed as the most humane and advanced level of interventive clinical social work" (Beaver and Miller, 1992, p. 353). Specifically, primary prevention is an advanced action aimed at forestalling or preventing a problem from occurring (see Table 7.1). Aimed at well or healthy elders, "practice at this level attempts to keep older people as physically, socially, and emotionally healthy as possible" (Schneider and Kropf, 1992, p. 4). Basically,

TABLE 7.1. Social Work Practice Focus and Roles in Three Levels of Prevention

	Primary Prevention	Secondary Prevention	Tertiary Prevention
Practice focus	Elder	Elder and informal caregivers	Elder, informal, and formal caregivers
Roles	Prevention	Maintenance	Rehabilitation
Enabler (empowerment)	1. Help spouse of terminally ill elder learn how to manage their bills and home.	1. Help elderly residents and family in a senior citizens apartment complex make decisions about how to increase safety awareness, thus preventing falls.	1. Help caregivers and nursing home residents decide on a strategy to include culturally sensitive foods on the menu or establish user-friendly visiting hours.
Broker	2. Link community elders to appropriate health-promoting water aerobics facilities that take into account gender or music preferences.	2. Link recently diagnosed diabetic and spouse to a community nutritionist with expertise in meal preparation and caloric intake to reduce obesity.	2. Link home-bound or institutionalized elder and informal caregiver with church to continue provision of communion or religious services.
Educator	3. Educate elders to share self-care strategies (tasty, low-fat, and salt-free recipes) in a brochure to be distributed at a senior center.	3. Educate family and elder regarding services available in an assisted-living facility.	3. Educate caregivers and elder about basic sign language techniques they can use with elders who have language impairments following a stroke.
Mediator	4. Negotiate conflict with employer and older worker in need of flex hours to care for spouse.	4. Negotiate conflict with home health care staff and elder regarding quality of services.	4. Negotiate conflict of family members selecting best nursing home for parent.
Coordinator	5. Coordinate high blood pressure screenings in nontraditional community-based settings, such as the church or beauty salon/barber shop.	5. Coordinate teenage-driven intergenerational volunteer program helping elders with chores, e.g., leaf and snow removal.	5. Coordinate services with American Red Cross to implement emergency response program with low-income and frail elders at home.

primary prevention includes two activities, health promotion and health protection, whose goal is to decrease the probability that elders will experience a "health-threatening event" (Kropf and Hutchison, 1992, p. 4).

For example, health promotion activities can increase the overall health of black Americans by increasing good health habits or disease prevention behaviors. Beaver and Miller (1992) suggest that "if people are careful about maintaining good dietary or nutritional standards throughout their lives, they may succeed in warding off the chronic conditions that characterize the aging process" (p. 33). Elders can be empowered to take control of their own health by teaching them ways to modify their risk factors (see Table 7.2). For instance, programs can teach aerobic/water exercises or how to prepare nutritional meals on a low budget, coupled with low-cholesterol and salt-free herbal recipes. Other activities to decrease the threat of a problem occurring include teaching elders how to accident-proof their homes or developing an elder-sensitive stop-smoking program.

Another type of primary intervention is specific protection for a particular group, such as African Americans. For example, older African Americans are at greater risk of kidney disease due to the high numbers diagnosed with hypertension. Primary health promotion programs can be developed to help African-American elders deal with the debilitating effects of high blood pressure by reducing their weight, exercising, and complying with medication regime and drug prescription (see Table 7.2). If the elderly engage in healthful practices on a sustained basis, debilitating and disabling conditions may be delayed or even avoided for the rest of their lives.

Secondary Prevention

Interventions at the secondary level are designed to begin with the onset of the problem, targeting early diagnosis and prompt treatment of a condition, both medical and social in nature (Beaver and Miller, 1992). Thus, an attempt is made to keep an acute problem from becoming chronic (Schneider and Kropf, 1992, p. 5). Relative to chronic health problems, one estimate is that five out of six people

TABLE 7.2. Health Risks and Preventive Care Among Older Blacks

Leading Preventable Causes of Death Among Older Black Adults	Modifiable Risk Factors
Heart diseases (cardiovascular) Stroke (cerebrovascular)	High blood pressure, high cholesterol levels, smoking, diabetes, diet, obesity, lack of exercise
Cancer	Smoking, diet, alcohol
Diabetes	Diet, obesity, alcohol, lack of exercise
Cirrhosis of the liver	Alcohol

Program Ideas

- Nutrition education (salt, sugar, cholesterol)

- Weight loss and control

- Exercise

- Smoking cessation

- Preventive services/screening especially for hypertension, diabetes, and prostate cancer and referral for alcohol abuse

- Stress management

Source: Adapted from American Association of Retired Persons, 1990a, p. 4.

over the age of sixty-five have at least one chronic health problem. Therefore, among black Americans, secondary prevention would be aimed toward elders who have started to manifest a problematic condition, such as diabetes. Black American elders and their families need to be empowered to address their secondary health needs and practices.

The major emphasis of secondary intervention, according to Beaver and Miller (1992), is to resolve problems to the greatest extent possible or to prevent more serious functional impairment, such as kidney failure, amputation, or blindness, among diabetic black American elders. Without proper treatment, these conditions can worsen. It is a known fact that black American elders are more likely to delay treatment than white elders when faced with increasing functional impairment (Harper, 1992).

As black Americans age, they frequently encounter social problems and experience greater losses that will put them at risk for social work intervention at this level. For instance, retirement is an event that many people anticipate with enjoyment. However, many black American elders face bleak retirement lives due to having fewer social opportunities and resources (Bureau of the Census, 1980; Gibson, 1988). Often, they have experienced a lifetime of low income and poverty, stemming from disadvantaged employment histories, such as low earnings from unskilled jobs, seasonal jobs, as well as limited medical insurance, pensions, and social security benefits. These handicapping work patterns over a lifetime have negative effects on the economic well-being of blacks as they reach old age (Abbott, 1980). Work in old age, in the same low-status jobs, becomes a necessity for many (Abbott, 1970). Social workers need to help black American elders with limited resources plan and develop effective and no-cost leisure activities to help them make a worthwhile transition into new and satisfying roles (MacNeil and Teague, 1987; Osgood, 1982).

Tertiary Prevention

The tertiary preventive or rehabilitative level of practice is aimed at impaired or frail elders in the community and those who are institutionalized. Specifically, tertiary interventions are aimed at ameliorating the effects of a dysfunctional condition (mental and/or physical) and helping elders regain as much of their functioning as possible (Beaver and Miller, 1992). At the tertiary level, social work involves empowering frail elders and their informal caregivers to join with formal helpers to provide comprehensive health care. Severely impaired and dependent elders will need to rely more on informal (family/friend) caregivers, supplemented by strong supports from formal agencies, to remain as independent as possible to the end of life (see Table 7.1).

Many families, including black Americans, provide community-based care for elders, even when they are severely impaired, to avoid institutionalization as long as possible (McGadney and Madison, 1997). Families, friends, and formal agencies provide supportive elder care, in that order (Taylor, 1985).

GERONTOLOGICAL SOCIAL WORK
INTERVENTIVE ROLES

In working with elders, their families, and formal caregivers, social workers are expected to be knowledgeable and skillful while filling a variety of interventive roles, utilizing a culturally sensitive multisystems approach of empowerment and collectivism. Compton and Galaway (1989) define an interventive role as a set of behaviors that both client and practitioner expect the practitioner to perform in an effort to fulfill the goals of the service contract. Each role identified in Table 7.1 has a different purpose with a client. Similarly, these roles can be undertaken at any practice level from primary to tertiary.

In the role of an *enabler,* Zastrow (1999) states that social workers "help individuals or groups to articulate their needs, clarify and identify their problems, explore resolution strategies, select and apply a strategy, and develop their capacities to deal with their own problems more effectively" (p. 18). In this role, social workers are encouraged to empower and enhance the lives of independent black American elders by encouraging and assisting them in using their internal strengths and coping mechanisms to solve their own problems more effectively. For example, at the primary level, Kropf and Hutchison (1992) suggest that social workers can discuss "with a recently widowed woman her fears about household management, such as paying bills or basic home maintenance, and expressing confidence in her ability to assume this responsibility once she learns the necessary procedures."

As a *broker,* geriatric social workers assess both environmental resources and client needs, thus linking elders who need help with appropriate services (Kropf and Hutchison, 1992). To be effective in this role, social workers must have both understanding and knowledge of the needs and resources of black American elders and the vast network of community services. At the tertiary level, for instance, an older black American caregiver of a severely retarded adult can be matched with a respite service so the two can attend weekly church services or in-home pastoral/missionary services can be facilitated. As another example, families of black American elders unable to continue living independently can be linked to an appropriate assisted-living or nursing facility.

An "*advocate* initiates action on behalf of a client . . . the practitioner takes the client's side and becomes a partisan spokesperson for an individual, group, or community" (Schneider and Kropf, 1992, p. 9). For example, an advocate can deal with specific situations, such as special needs of patients in long-term care facilities (particularly nursing homes). Also, in a senior center building, practitioners can assist elders in negotiating with the senior center staff to have a no-smoking section for a group of nonsmoking participants at the primary level of practice (Kropf and Hutchison, 1992).

In the role of *educator,* social workers have the potential to impart information about health standards and effective health practices to a wide variety of black American elders before a condition is manifest. This can include a variety of activities, such as participating in leadership seminars, making appearances on television and radio, and writing articles for newspapers, magazines, journals, or other publications. For instance, at the secondary level, a group of volunteers can be taught how to staff a telephone reassurance system for diabetic elders. Also, at the primary level, well elders can be educated about the benefits of using stress management to maintain good health.

The *mediator* role for social workers involves intervention in disputes between parties to help them find compromises, reconcile differences, or reach mutually satisfactory agreements. At the secondary level, for example, practitioners can discuss and clarify menu complaints with staff and participants of a home-delivered meal program (Kropf and Hutchison, 1992).

As *coordinators,* social workers bring components together in an organized manner. Zastrow (1999) coordinated at the tertiary level with a nutritionist with expertise in low-salt meal preparation to give a lecture series, including demonstrations to staff in a nursing home, to help in the development of culturally sensitive meals for elders with high blood pressure.

BARRIERS

Despite the effectiveness of these intervention roles, a major public health challenge is to effectively target primary prevention efforts at African-American elders—mounting highly efficient intervention efforts. Thus, barriers to risk reduction will include the linguistic and cultural diversity of the population, low levels of income and education, and the fact that a high proportion of African Americans tend to live in physical and social environments that do not reinforce positive health choices (see Table 7.3). Barriers to primary prevention behaviors, particularly barriers related to socioeconomic status, need to be identified so that culturally appropriate interventions can be developed. The deficits of African-American males, particularly the elderly, have important ramifications for family structure and economic status, and, thereby, an indirect effect on health status. In addition, the numbers of poor elderly African-American women are likely to increase (Beckles, Blount, and Jiles, 1994).

CONCLUSION

The burden of chronic disease is likely to increase among black elders if the current levels of risk prevail. A major challenge for social workers is to effectively target primary prevention efforts at black American elders. They must recognize the heterogeneity of black elders, identify behaviors that protect their health, and design intervention and health promotion activities that reinforce positive self-care behaviors. Also, social workers must recognize that barriers to primary prevention and risk reduction will include the linguistic and cultural diversity of the black elderly population, low levels of income and education, and the fact that a high proportion live in physical and social environments that do not reinforce positive health choices. Appropriate interventions can be developed if these barriers are identified. In keeping with the collectivism approach to practice, successful outcomes include the collaborative and mutual involvement of black elders and their families.

TABLE 7.3. Barriers to Utilization of Health Promotion/Prevention Services by Black American Elders

---

Ageism
- Individualized elder services neglected
- Age disparity between client and provider
- Negative attitudes about aging processes
- Lack of knowledge about normal aging processes

Physical Access to Services
- Transportation inadequate
- Location of facilities and programs
- Rural access issues
- Lack of physicians willing to accept Medicaid patients
- Lack of trained minority professionals

Economic Access to Services
- Poverty among black Americans
- Lack of insurance coverage
- Lack of funds for copayment
- Lack of physicians who will accept Medicaid patients

Cultural Access to Services
- Inadequate outreach to black American elders
- Language barriers/lack of bicultural staff
- Lack of culturally sensitive services
- Underrepresentation of black American health providers in community
- Lack of familiarity with bureaucracies
- Historically experienced discrimination and oppression
- Distrust of service providers
- Stigma associated with admitting a need or using public programs
- Knowledge of services
- Inequalities in the health care services
- Limited use of lay consultants
- Knowledge of illness/disease
- Education materials not culturally sensitive

Source: Adapted from Schoenrock, 1990; Tarnove, 1992, pp. 24-26.

REFERENCES

Abbott, J. (1970). Socioeconomic characteristics of the elderly: Some black/white differences. *Social Security Bulletin, 40*(1), 16-42.

Abbott, J. (1980). Work experience and earnings of middle-aged black and white men, 1965-1971. *Social Security Bulletin, 43*(12), 16-34.

American Association of Retired Persons (1990a). *Healthy aging: Making health promotion work for minority elders.* Washington, DC: AARP National Resource Center on Health Promotion and Aging, AARP Health Advocacy Series.

American Association of Retired Persons (1990b). *A portrait of older minorities.* Washington, DC: American Association of Retired Persons, Minority Affairs Initiatives.

Angel, J. and Hogan, D. (1994). The demography of minority aging populations. In *Minority elders: Five goals toward building a public policy base* (Second edition) (pp. 9-21). Washington, DC: Gerontological Society of America.

Baker, F.M. (1988). Dementing illness and black Americans. In J.S. Jackson, P. Newton, A. Ostfield, D. Savage, and E.L. Schneider (Eds.), *The black American elderly: Research on physical and psychosocial health* (pp. 215-233). New York: Springer.

Beaver, M.L. and Miller, D.A. (1992). *Clinical social work practice with the elderly: Primary, secondary, and tertiary intervention* (Second edition). Belmont, CA: Wadsworth Publishing Company.

Beckles, L.A., Blount, S.B., and Jiles, R.B. (1994). African American. In N.L. Keenan (Ed.), *Chronic disease in minority populations: African-Americans, American Indians and Alaska Natives, Asians and Pacific Islanders, Hispanic Americans* (pp. 1-34).U.S. Department of Health and Human Services, Public Health Service, Centers for Disease Control and Prevention, National Center for Chronic Disease Prevention and Health Promotion. Atlanta, GA: Office of Surveillance and Analysis.

Bureau of the Census (1980). *The social and economic status of the black population.* Current Population Reports, Special Studies P-23, No. 80. Washington, DC: U.S. Department of Commerce.

Centers for Disease Control (1992). *Behavioral Risk Factor Surveillance System, 1991-1992* (pp. 8-26). Atlanta, GA: Office of Surveillance and Analysis.

Clayton, L.A. and Byrd, W.M. (1993). The African-American cancer crisis, part I: The problem. *Journal of Health Care for the Poor and Underserved, 4*(2), 83-101.

Cochran, D. and McGadney, B.F. (1997). *It takes a village: A multi-system approach to preventing hypertension among older African Americans.* Paper presented at the 15th Anniversary Conference of the Association for Gerontology and Human Development in Historically Black Colleges and Universities, Tampa, FL.

Compton, B.R. and Galaway, B. (1989). *Social work processes* (Fourth edition). Homewood, IL: Dorsey Press.

Davis, L. and Maryland, M. (1997). Health promotion: The mature years (64 and older). In K.M. Allen and J.M. Phillips (Eds.), *Women's health across the life span: A comprehensive perspective* (pp. 89-101). New York: Lippincott Company.

Davis, L. and McGadney, B.F. (1993). Self-care practices of black elders. In C.M. Barresi and D.E. Stull (Eds.), *Ethnic elderly and long-term care* (pp. 97-107). New York: Springer Publishing Company.

Davis, L., McGadney, B.F., and Perri, P.K. (1990a). *Living with arthritis: A self-care guide for black elders.* Lisle, IL: Tucker Publishing Company.

Davis, L., McGadney, B.F., and Perri, P.K. (1990b). *Living with diabetes: A self-care guide for black elders.* Lisle, IL: Tucker Publishing Company.

Davis, L., McGadney, B.F., and Perri, P.K. (1990c). *Living with hypertension: A self-care guide for black elders.* Lisle, IL: Tucker Publishing Company.

Dilworth-Anderson, P. (1992). Extended kin networks in black families. *Families in Aging, 17*(Summer), 29-32.

Gibson, R.C. (1988). The work, retirement, and disability of older black Americans. In J.S. Jackson (Ed.), *The black elderly: Research on physical and psychosocial health* (pp. 304-326). New York: Springer Publishing Company.

Harper, M.S. (1992). Elderly issues in the African-American community. In R.L. Braithwaite and S.E. Taylor (Eds.), *Health issues in the black community* (pp. 222-238). San Francisco: Jossey-Bass.

Kropf, N.P. and Hutchison, E.D. (1992). Effective practice with elderly clients. In R.L. Schneider and N.P. Kropf (Eds.), *Gerontological social work: Knowledge, service settings, and special populations.* Chicago: Nelson-Hall Publishers.

MacNeil, R.D. and Teague, M.L. (1987). *Aging and leisure: Vitality in later life.* Englewood Cliffs, NJ: Prentice-Hall.

McGadney, B.F. (1992). Stressors and social supports as predictors of burden for black and white caregivers of elders with dementia. Unpublished dissertation. Chicago, IL: The University of Chicago.

McGadney, B.F. (1995). Family, church, and formal social supports of African American caregivers of impaired elders. In R.J. Taylor (Ed.), *African American research perspectives* (pp. 34-44). Ann Arbor, MI: University of Michigan, Institute for Social Research (ISR).

McGadney, B.F. and Madison, A. (1997). Use of formal community services by family caregivers of African American elders. *Michigan Academician, 29,* 199-220.

Miller, B.A., Ries, L.A.G., Hankey, B.F., Kosary, C.L., Harras, A., Devesa, S.S., and Edwards, B.K. (Eds.) (1990). *SEER Cancer Statistics Review: 1973-1990.* DHHS publication no. (NIH)93-2789. Bethesda, MD: National Cancer Institute.

National Center for Health Statistics (1992). *Health, United States.* DHHS publication no. (PHS)93-1232. Hyattsville, MD: National Center for Health Statistics.

O'Brien, T.R., Flanders, W.D., Decoufle, P., Boyle, C.A., DeStefano, F., and Teutsch, S. (1989). Are racial differences in the prevalence of diabetes in adults explained by differences in obesity? *Journal of the American Medical Association, 262,* 1485-1488.

Osgood, N. (1982). *Life after work: Retirement, leisure, recreation and the elderly.* New York: Praeger.

Otten, M., Teutsch, S.M., Williamson, D.F., and Marks, J.S. (1990). The effect of known risk factors on the excess mortality of black adults in the United States. *JAMA, 263*(6), 845-850.

Pappas, G., Queen, S., Hadden, W., and Fisher, G. (1993). The increasing disparity between socioeconomic groups in the United States, 1960 and 1986. *New England Journal of Medicine, 329*(2), 103-109.

Polednak, A.P. (1989). *Racial and ethnic differences in disease.* New York: Oxford University Press.

Potter, L.B. (1991). Socioeconomic determinants of white and black males' life expectancy differentials, 1980. *Demography, 28*(2), 303-321.

Public Health Service (1991a). *Healthy people 2000: National health promotion and disease prevention objectives, 1991.* DHHS publication no. (PHS) 91-50212. Washington, DC: U.S. Government Printing Office.

Public Health Service. (1991b). The nation's health: Special populations. In *Healthy people 2000: National health promotion and disease prevention objectives, 1991* (pp. 594-605). DHHS publication no. (PHS) 91-50212. Washington, DC: U.S. Government Printing Office.

Public Health Service (1993). *Health, United States 1992, 1993.* (DHHS publication no. (PHS) 93-1232:49. Washington, DC: U.S. Government Printing Office.

Rogers, R.G. (1992). Living and dying in the U.S.A.: Sociodemographic determinants of death among blacks and whites. *Demography, 29*(2), 287-303.

Schneider, R.L. and Kropf, N.P. (Eds.) (1992). *Gerontological social work: Knowledge, service settings, and special populations.* Chicago: Nelson-Hall Publishers.

Schoenrock, S.A. (1990). *Health education and promotion among multicultural populations.* Publisher # HE: 1002:M91. San Diego, CA: National Resource Center on Minority Aging Populations.

Sorlie, P., Rogot, E., Anderson, R., Johnson, N.J., and Backlund, E. (1992). *Lancet, 340*(August 8), 346-350.

Tarnove, L. (1992). Delivery of health promotion programs: Outreach to minority elders. pp. 24-26. Washington, DC: AARP: National Eldercare Institute on Health Promotion.

Taylor, R.J. (1985). The extended family as a source of support to elderly African Americans. *The Gerontologist, 25,* 488-495.

Truman, B.I., Lentzner, H.R., Keenan, N.L., and Harris, J.R. (1994). Introduction. In N.L. Keenan (Ed.), *Chronic disease in minority populations: African-Americans, American Indians and Alaska Natives, Asians and Pacific Islanders, Hispanic Americans* (pp. 1-5). U.S. Department of Health and Human Services, Public Health Service, Centers for Disease Control and Prevention, National Center for Chronic Disease Prevention and Health Promotion. Atlanta, GA: Office of Surveillance and Analysis.

Wykle, M. and Kaskel, B. (1994). Increasing the longevity of minority older adults through improved health status. In *Minority elders: Five goals toward building a public policy base* (pp. 32-39). Washington, DC: The Gerontological Society of America.

Zarit, S.H. (1980). *Aging and mental disorders.* New York: Macmillan.

Zastrow, C.H. (1999). *The practice of social work* (Sixth edition). Pacific, CA: Brooks/Cole Publishing.

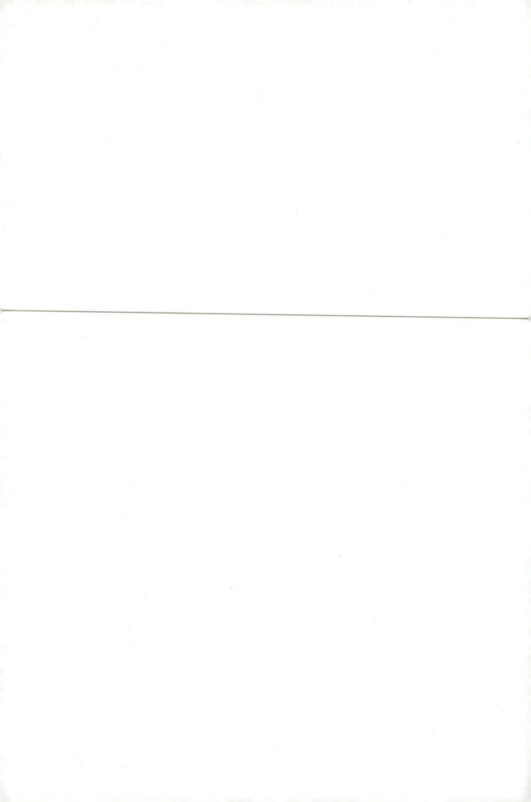

PART III:
SELF-HEALING, COLLECTIVISM,
AND SOCIAL ACTION
IN THE BLACK COMMUNITY:
FORMAL AND INFORMAL HELPING

Chapter 8

African-Centered Reality Therapy: Intervention and Prevention

Elijah Mickel

INTRODUCTION

African-centered reality therapy is presented as a viable alternative for those who wish to consider a different way to work with the African-American family. This approach is designed to prevent disequilibrium and, when it occurs, to restore balance. It is an approach for intervention and prevention. To improve intervention and prevention, we must expand our vision of the family. The social work profession has a traditional philosophical and practice foundation based on individualization and dependence. Using the concepts that are implicit to individual-focused models, practitioners, although claiming a strengths perspective, continue to label families. These labels are generally pathological and non-need fulfilling. This has allowed those who practice to blame the victims, resulting in family destabilization.

For the purpose of this chapter, intervention is the process of teaching families to meet their needs in a responsible manner. Families meet their needs responsibly when their need-fulfilling behaviors do not interfere with those outside the family structure. Prevention is the process of expanding the helping environment so that it includes the total family environment. Included in the concept of total family environment are family thoughts, feelings, actions, and its physical structure. The total family environment is composed of the internal and the external task environment. The task environment (Thompson, 1967) includes the components that are perceived by the family as necessary for need fulfillment. The nurturing environment is where the family and the practitioner interface to develop a need-fulfilling helping environment. This includes a spiritually, physically, and mentally comfortable situation.

PURPOSE

The purpose of this chapter is to provide a foundation for further inquiry while expanding the base of social work practice with families. This chapter builds a treatment platform from which to create an architectural foundation for understanding the black family. This platform provides the necessary transparency for expanding African-centered reality therapy into the non-African community. Integrating African-centered reality therapy into our family practice expands the available theoretical and practice base for professionals. Practitioners have worked with African-American families and, as a result, have developed some best-practice methods without developing a new paradigm. They have presented methods—some that are effective—but have not restructured their intervention specifically for practice in the African-American community. This chapter is an attempt to change our way of addressing therapeutic intervention. According to Minnich (1990), "Such changes are necessary, I believe, not only to transform what is accepted as knowledge by the dominant culture and what is passed on to new generations, but for the sake of thinking itself. We cannot think well as long as we are locked into old errors that are so familiar as to be virtually invisible" (p. 1).

What is good for the oppressed is usually very good for those who are not oppressed. The very nature of the inquiry provides a discourse that will, in the final analysis, help families and the profession.

CHOICE THEORY
AND AFRICAN-CENTERED REALITY THERAPY

Reality therapy (RT), developed by Dr. William Glasser (1965), is a process that teaches people a better way to fulfill their needs

(Glasser, 1980). It is a way to gain and maintain a successful identity. The Institute for Reality Therapy (IRT) *Policies and Procedures Manual* (1987, p. 22) defines reality therapy as "an approach to counseling, educating and living which continues to be developed. The principles of this approach are totally consistent with the concepts of control theory." This method has two major components: the counseling (nurturing or helping) environment and the procedures that lead to change (Mickel, 1993).

The IRT *Policies and Procedures Manual* (1987) defines control theory as

> [a] biological theory which explains why and how all living organisms behave. All any organism can do is behave and all behaviors are total. Every total behavior is always the organism's best attempt to meet its basic needs. All total behaviors are internally motivated and purposeful. We are genetically instructed to live our lives in ways which will allow us to meet our basic needs. (p. 35)

Choice theory (CT) (Glasser, 1996, 1998) posits that all human beings have five basic needs—one physiological (survival) and four psychological. Most of us would concur on the need for survival. The four psychological needs are love, power, fun, and freedom.

1. *Love* or belonging is a basic need reflected in a need to love and be loved. We all need at least one significant image in our lives. Glasser's (1988, p. 3) definition of love and belonging is "to gain and maintain the belief that others whom we care for are concerned enough about us so that they will both give us and accept from us the affection, care and friendship we desire."
2. *Power* is the sense of worth and worthiness—to feel good and have others feel good about you, as Glasser (1988, p. 3) states, "to gain and maintain the belief that we are recognized by some others some of the time as having something to do or say that they believe and we agree is important."
3. *Fun* is a need to do that which you wish to do simply because you enjoy it. Glasser (1988, p. 3) states, "to gain and maintain the belief that we are having fun, we must engage in some

behavior that has (for its main purpose) enjoyment and in which there is laughter and good feeling on the part of all involved."

4. *Freedom* involves the ability to choose, to come or go within the environment. Simply put, it is the process of making choices. As Glasser (1988, p. 3) states, freedom means "to gain and maintain the belief that we can act and think without restriction by others as long as we do not significantly interfere with their access to the same freedom we desire."

These basic needs are the determinants of all behavior, although one essential African-centered component is missing, spirituality.

Spirituality

African-centered reality therapy/choice theory (Mickel, 1991) adds another dimension to these basic needs. That missing component is spirituality (see Figure 8.1). Spirituality (Ani, 1994; Mbiti, 1969; Mickel, 1991; Somé, 1993) is essential to the process of moving to a holistic model of intervention and prevention. African-centered reality therapy reaffirms and incorporates the need for spirituality as essential to holism. A number of authors have defined spirituality as the foundation for effective practice. Spirituality is the process of knowing without knowing how or why we know; it is our connection to the Divine; it provides the answer to the unanswerable. Spirituality makes the invisible visible. Spirituality includes the quest for personal meaning and relationships that are beyond mind and body. It is the interconnectiveness between the living and the "many thousands gone." According to Cornett (1992), "A definition of spirituality would need to broadly encompass the individual's understanding of and response to meaning in life; time and mortality; expectations regarding what, if anything, follows death; and belief or nonbelief in a 'higher power'" (p. 101).

The practice of developing a relationship in the helping professions is itself spiritual (Canda, 1988). A cursory review of the African-centered literature (Asante, 1988; Asante and Asante, 1990; Azibo, 1989; Baldwin, 1986; Carruthers, 1980; Fanon, 1967; Karenga, 1984, 1989, 1990; Richards, 1990; Semmes, 1981) presents spirituality as a template, a litmus test for a holistic life. According

FIGURE 8.1. Intervention and Prevention: African-Centered Reality Therapy

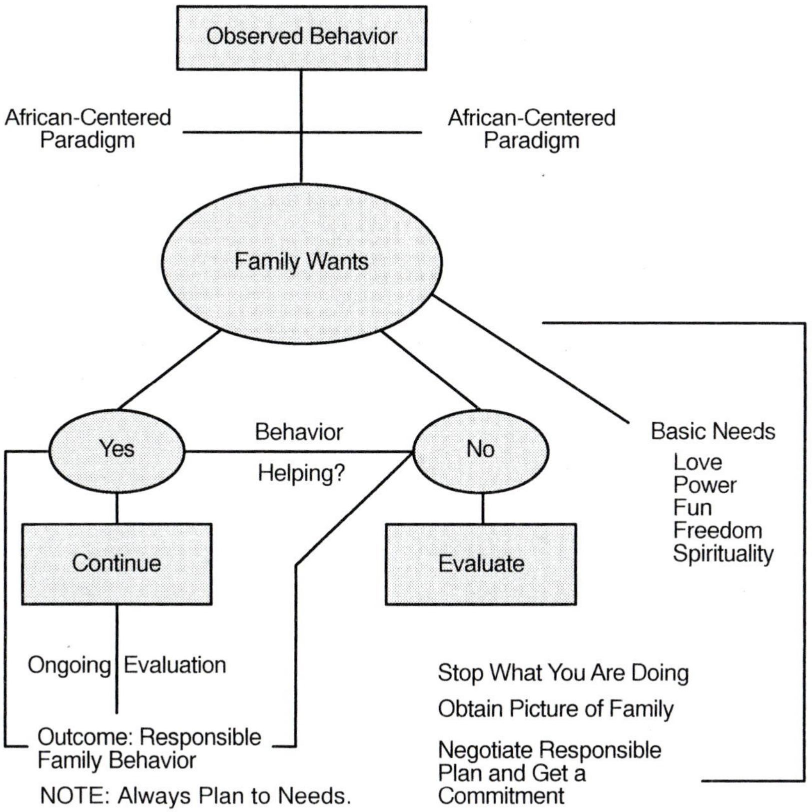

to Asante (1988), "You are its ultimate test. You test its authenticity by incorporating it into your behavior. At the apex of your consciousness, it becomes your life because everything you do, it is (p. 6)." Spirituality is expressed as both views and behavior. It is transcendence and a basic human characteristic. It expresses a sense of relatedness to something greater than self (Beckett and Johnson, 1995). Spirituality is a scale upon which we weigh the worthiness of an approach or process as it applies to the family. Theoretical and practical approaches are incomplete if they fail to consider spirituality as an essential component.

African-Centered Paradigm

The African-centered approach joins traditional cultural values that are over 2,000 years old (Ani, 1994; Budge, 1960; Karenga, 1984, 1989, 1990; Massey, 1970) with choice theory. It approaches human behavior from a different perspective than the Eurocentric model. The Eurocentric model posits that a clear separation exists between the individual and society. A split exists between mind and body, with the emphasis on the individual rather than on groupings of individuals or relations among individuals (Joseph, Reddy, and Searle-Chatterjee, 1990). African-centered reality therapy can be used to liberate the family from the limits of the constricting Eurocentric environment. As suggested by Fanon (1967), "Thus human reality in-itself-for-itself can be achieved only through conflict and through the risk that conflict implies. This risk means that I go beyond life toward a supreme good that is the transformation of subjective certainty of my own worth into a universally valid objective truth" (p. 218). The universally valid objective truth, from an African-centered perspective, is manifested in the family. African-centered RT/CT provides a method by which the family is empowered. Families are provided an opportunity to increase perceptual choices while maintaining a harmonious relationship within their perceptual world.

The African-centered approach is grounded in the basic principles of human personality based upon the following traditional African beliefs:

1. The divine image of humans
2. The perfectibility of humans
3. The teachability of humans
4. Free will of humans
5. The essentiality of moral social practice (Karenga, 1990)

The African-centered approach also includes the following seven principles (*Nguzo Saba*). The *Nguzo Saba* (Karenga, 1989) interpret and guide the African-centered personality in daily living:

1. *Umoja* (unity)
2. *Kujichagulia* (free will/self-determination)
3. *Ujima* (helping one another)
4. *Ujamaa* (buying goods and services from one another)
5. *Nia* (purpose)
6. *Kuumba* (creativity)
7. *Imani* (spirituality)

The seven hermetic principles (Three Initiates, 1988) are the philosophical underpinning for understanding the ancient African worldview:

1. Correspondence
2. Gender
3. Cause/effect
4. Vibration
5. Rhythm
6. Polarity
7. Mentalism

Practitioners must move from the philosophical to the practical. In this move, the human personality must guide the practice. The entity known as the human personality is the result of the culmination of many components that are expressed as our behavior. This entity is built upon our values, knowledge, and sensory inputs, and is guided by our basic needs. The values, knowledge, and sensory inputs result in perception. The human personality requires relationships. Therefore, relationships and the resultant interconnections provide the parameters for subsequent practice. The human personality results from our perception of the world. The values and knowledge along with our sensory system guide the behavioral choices made. Perception guides the behavioral choices that are selected while behavior attempts to control perception.

The African-centered matrix correlates the relationship between the philosophical principles and the basic needs (see Table 8.1). This matrix provides a sense of wholeness when used to guide our understanding of the African worldview that is the underpinning.

*Essentiality of Moral Social Practice—Love—*Umoja*—Correspondence/Gender*

Correspondence is a principle that describes relationships. Whatever occurs within the family affects actions outside the family. Whatever occurs with the parent/caregiver affects the children. Whatever affects the living affects those to be born. According to the Three Initiates (1988, p. 24):

> There are planes beyond our knowing, but when we apply the Principle of Correspondence to them we are able to understand much that would otherwise be unknowable to us. This Principle is of universal application and manifestation, on the various planes of the material, mental, and spiritual universe—it is a Universal Law. The ancient Hermetists considered this Principle as one of the most important mental instruments by which man was able to pry aside the obstacles which hid from view the Unknown.

Gender is a principle that describes creation. It is manifested at all levels and seen in the union of opposites. Within the family structure, a process of creation provides for the continuation of the family structure. What may be most akin to this principle is the construct of negative entropy. Negative entropy posits that all living organisms must take in more energy than they require to exist. Gender exists on

TABLE 8.1. African-Centered Matrix

Philosophy	Basic Needs	*Nguzo Saba*	Hermetic
Essentiality of Moral Social Practice	Love	*Umoja*	Correspondence Gender
Free Will	Freedom	*Kujichagulia*	Cause/Effect
Perfectibility	Power	*Ujima/Nia/Ujamaa*	Vibration/Rhythm
Teachability	Fun	*Kuumba*	Polarity
Divine Image	Spirituality	*Imani*	Mentalism

all levels and is seen within the family structure when one evaluates the use to which the energy, necessary for the continuation of the structure, is put. According to the Three Initiates (1988, p. 148), "The office of Gender is solely that of creating, producing, generating, etc., and its manifestations are visible on every plane of phenomena."

The essentiality of moral social practice posits that good is that which lasts and uplifts families. It charges people with making the world a better place in which to live. Moral social practice is essential to the well-being of all humanity and guides our practice. Families share responsibility not only for themselves but for the entire village and must all work for the good of humanity. The move toward self-actualization is seen in the family's relation to the community and how it perceives itself in this relationship. This concept reaffirms that we are all one humanity and that the only good that is done is that which is done for those who need it. It is the unifying principle that cements and provides the foundation on which to build responsibility to act responsibly in the real world.

Umoja (unity) is especially pertinent to the African-centered family since it has no divisions in its structure, except those which are artificially created in the Eurocentric consciousness. There are no individuals, only unions within families and communities. To be family is to be a part of a whole that requires sharing family responsibilities. It means sharing the joy as well as the tribulations that come to a body that is conceptually a single unit. There are no outer limits to membership nor are there limits on family or community obligation. The family is the unit from which we can receive all of our basic needs, and it can be the most need-fulfilling environment. Family is solidified as is required by a moral imperative. The family creates the structure required to develop energy for its continued existence. Its foundation is love and belonging that requires collective unity.

Unity is the process of placing the needs of the family above wants of the individual. The parameters of individuals are defined within the family and are inextricably bound to the collective. Individuals lose their identity when they perceive themselves as separate from the family. *Umoja* reflects the family's vision in its communal struggle for inclusion. The practitioner can discern the vision through an understanding of the interrelationship of the essentiality of moral social practice, love, and belonging, *Umoja,* and correspondence and gender.

Free Will—Freedom—**Kujichagulia**—*Cause/Effect*

Families that take control of their destiny are actors rather than reactors. The members plan their lives to be choosers and not controlled. The Three Initiates (1988, p. 144) reveal:

> The majority of people are carried along like the falling stone, obedient to environment, outside influences and internal moods, desires, etc., not to speak of the desires and wills of others stronger than themselves, heredity, environment, and suggestion, carrying them along without resistance on their part, or the exercise of the Will. Moved like the pawns on the checkerboard of life, they play their parts and are laid aside after the game is over.

Under the auspices of the African-centered matrix, the family is viewed as having choice. The members approach life from differing points of view. They see themselves as problem solvers. Time is a tool that is useful for effective intervention.

Free will means that families have choice. Choice may be constrained by lack of information. People have options when they take action. Free will is grounded in moral conscience, and people will make responsible choices when they have information and values that lead them in that direction. Knowledge and values are essential to informed free-will decisions. Together they form an integral part of the perceptual system and, thus, significantly affect subsequent behaviors. Behavior is organized around the control of perceptions. All that anyone can do is behave. There are natural laws, and free will allows one to choose healthy need-fulfilling behaviors. All behavior is motivated by our basic needs and follows the natural laws.

The family that practices self-determination knows its history and the history of its community. *Kujichagulia* (self-determination) is, in essence, the ability to describe and name oneself. Self-determination further connects families with their ancestors and traditions. *Kujichagulia* is reflected by the family's choosing to view its behavior as healthy rather than pathological. The role of the practitioner is then one of understanding the choices families make and framing intervention that is appropriate to those choices. In times of trouble and distress, the family will fall back upon its strength-fulfilling behaviors and look within them for answers to present problems. African-American families have solved their problems based on traditional knowledge and values. These traditions have become family rituals. Rituals are behaviors that are unique to a family and utilized to deal with perceived problems. It is necessary to do a family historical analysis to ascertain how ritual history influences family choices. Utilizing the African-centered approach, it is important that practitioners understand the meaning of rituals and their relevance to the presenting problem.

The issue of self-determination is also an issue of control. All families have the need to be self-determining, and when that need is thwarted, they behave to fulfill this need. Thus, when families (whatever defines that family—class, culture, choice, membership, ethnicity) are denied self-determination (freedom and power) their behavior will reflect the unfilled need. Families do what they do to meet their basic needs as they are viewed through *Kujichagulia.*

*Perfectibility—Power—*Ujima/Nia/Ujamaa—*Vibration/Rhythm*

The principle of vibration teaches us that the rate of change or motion within families differs. Family behavior is described by its rate of movement or change—that, in fact, the family is never constant but always in a state of motion. The rate and range of this motion and its subsequent impact varies with different family systems; it also varies within different subsystems. The African family is not a monolithic structure, even when it appears to be so. There is an interrelationship and interconnectedness within families. This is known as "familiness," which manifests itself in the collective consciousness of the family. According to the Three Initiates' (1988, p. 115), "They [the family] teach that all manifestations of thought, emotion, reason, will or desire, or any mental state or condition, are accompanied by vibrations, a portion of which are thrown off and which tend to affect the minds of other persons by 'induction.'"

The principle of rhythm deals with the epigenetic development of the family structure. Mickel (1990, p. 30) relates, "Developmentally, family members move from simple role functions to complex ones. Members perform relatively simple processes in the early stages of their family involvement and are reared with the expectation that they can take on more complex functions as they develop." Family structure moves from undifferentiated to differentiation. The African family has rhythm. When the practitioner studies the family, he or she can discern its rhythm. According to the Three Initiates (1988, p. 129), "Thus it is with all living things; they are born, grow and die—and then are reborn. So it is with all great movements, philosophies, creeds, fashions, governments, nations and all else— birth, growth, maturity, decadence, death—and then new birth." When one focuses upon rhythm, one is able to effectively assess the family's development.

The perfectibility of humans posits that there is continuous development. This principle suggests that humans develop progressively and are perpetually becoming. It is through this process that they move to the possibility of assimilation with the "higher power." There is a focus upon the spiritual development of the human being. This philosophical position reifies progress within the family structure, and it is understood that children have the possibility of becoming better than their parents if they "do the right thing." Growth occurs in the physical as well as in a spiritual sense. We must never forget that a holistic perspective demands that we look at growth and development on the spiritual plane as well as the physical or mental. Again, this principle undergirds the work that practitioners do with their clients, as it reinforces the actuality of movement from irresponsibility to responsibility. Perfectibility provides a rationale for using African-centered reality therapy/choice theory, and this is our purpose.

There is no more empowering concept than purpose (*Nia*). Among families there appears no more intense drive than the search for purpose. A key component of family self-awareness is the sense of *Nia*. The knowledge of what I am depends upon knowledge of who we are. Who we are depends upon knowing our history and our role in the continuation of the family's growth and development.

In the reality therapy/choice theory approach, purpose can be assessed through our pictures. The pictures that we form in our head become the impetus or purpose for our behavior. Pictures are purpose, and purpose is defined by our pictures. Thus, when we attempt to match pictures, we are matching purpose from the perspective of the African-centered matrix.

Purpose allows one to be generous in prosperity. Prosperity is viewed as a blessing and when one is blessed, one has an obligation to help those who are in need. When confronted with someone who is in need, families believe that it is their obligation to share their blessings. It is through our understanding of *Ujima* (helping one another) that we work to build and contribute more than those who came before us. We begin to think new thoughts and relate to the world and ourselves in a different way.

The objective is to develop the necessary resources to be self-sufficient. The self-sufficient family comes to the collective world with something of worth to offer. An emphasis upon building internal resources is essential to the family sustaining itself in the area of providing survival needs. *Ujamaa* (buying goods and services from one another) is the foundation of the community from an economic perspective that is based upon sharing and meeting the needs of the community.

*Teachability—Fun—*Kuumba*—Polarity*

The principle that all behavior exists on a continuum provides another strong rationale for intervention in the family system. If one understands the presenting problem, the solution is also near. All problems as well as solutions should be viewed on a continuum. Every problem has a solution, and this solution is inherent to the problem. Just as health and illness are interdependent, existing on the same continuum, one cannot exist without the other. According to the Three Initiates (1988, p. 125), "Everything is dual; everything has poles; everything has its pair of opposites; like and unlike are the same; opposites are identical in nature, but different in degree; extremes meet; all truths are but half-truths; all paradoxes may be reconciled."

The teachability of humans posits that people are teachable and capable of moral cultivation that leads to their higher selves. The goal of teaching is wisdom based upon morality. Morality is defined by the family and community within which one is living. A theoretical underpinning that promotes the use of the African-centered reality therapy/choice theory-based intervention becomes viable from the frame of reference of teachability of its clients. This model recognizes the value of information/knowledge as a key process in choosing behavior (which, after all, is based upon perception).

Kuumba (creativity) is the essential component in restoration, healing, and repairing oppressed people. They, creatively, fashion a way of coping within a rejecting society. It is through this process that we restructure our world. We use the African-centered creative process to change misinformation and develop a new history. According to Asante (1988, p. 6), "Afrocentricity is the belief in the centrality of Africans in postmodern history. It is our history, our mythology, our creative motif, and our ethos exemplifying our collective will. On basis of our story, we build upon the work of our ancestors who gave signs toward our humanizing function."

The creative aspect of the *Nguzo Saba* is the organization/reorganizational aspect of choice theory. When we are confronted by barriers to our continued homeostasis, we then must attempt to use available resources to alter our behavior. If resources are not available to solve or resolve the problems, we must use our creativity to develop some. Creativity is the celebration of the Good as it presents life as an opportunity and challenge. Life is worth living, and we must struggle for liberation, victory, love for one another, vision, values, and the right to make our own decisions.

Divine Image—Spirituality—Imani—Mentalism

Families, through mentalism, bring their being into existence, and they, through the process of creation, begin the cycle of events that unify the past and the future. It is through the creation of a mental picture turned into action behaviors that the divine image, the spiritual need, and *Imani* are fulfilled. The family is the locus for the development of controlled change. The parameters that are erected by the family add to the interconnectiveness of the members over time. According to the Three Initiates (1988, p. 43):

Under and behind all outward appearances or manifestations, there must always be a substantial Reality. This is the Law. Man considering the Universe, of which he is a unit, sees nothing but change in matter, forces, and mental states. He sees that nothing really IS, but that everything is BECOMING and CHANGING.

The belief of divine image posits that one is born in the context of possibility and that errors can be corrected through teaching and subsequent self-corrective practices. This belief is the essence of what one does as a therapist—persons can choose to change if they obtain enough information. It provides the foundation upon which intervention is built. To intervene, one must believe that it will result in a possibility of positive change.

Spirituality takes the position that one has a spiritual self. This spiritual self is the higher one and belongs to a different plane, whereas the physical self belongs to the earth. It is within this principle that one who wishes to work with the African-American family begins to understand the presentation of spiritual needs as distinct and as powerful as the other basic needs.

Imani (faith) suggests that we must believe in ourselves and our humanity so that we can be in harmonious/natural order with the universe. We must have the faith, to have the consciousness to investigate, delineate, and invigorate our families and those who are of a like mind. This model posits that there is perfectibility and teachability. Faith reaffirms our past glory and greatness in our future.

Spirituality, *Imani*, mentalism, and divine image of humans are people centered, suggesting that if one is to be successful with intervention, one must begin where the person starts. Spirituality posits that one cannot work, holistically, without including the mind, body, and spirit in the change process. Any analysis of this position includes an understanding that irresponsibility is in direct conflict with these principles. The African-centered paradigm takes a position that one has an obligation to oneself as well as to others. A people that cannot save itself is destined to remain enslaved forever. We must set our own standards based upon the expectations for success.

Reality Therapy

Case Study

The following case was sent to a special unit (voluntary care). The voluntary care unit, a component of foster care services in a public welfare department, was designed to work with families and children in short-term placement. The unit was the provider of a continuum of care from intake though permanent placement. The goal was family preservation, while the objective was to reduce the time in foster care for children placed in voluntary care. Placements could last no longer than 120 days and were strictly voluntary. The foundation of this unit developed from what was then an alternative paradigm. The unit was founded on an African-centered view of the family. Cases were processed with an understanding that the family was a self-defined entity. It was more than the blood relations as defined in the foster care regulations. In fact, the unit placed children with "kin" and surrogate parents. It had even placed with "play" parents/relatives.

> A mother was self-referred and requested temporary foster care for her six-year-old son. She related that she was having emotional problems and was not able to continue to care safely for her child. She had obtained a statement from her general practitioner to this effect. It was explained that temporary foster care had a four-month limit. The mother related that she would be well at the end of the four months.
>
> To accept the child, the agency required as much information, on all relatives and friends who might be potential caregivers, as could be gathered. According to the mother, no relatives or friends were available to care for this child. The father's whereabouts were reportedly unknown. The mother was an only child. The maternal grandmother refused to care for the child, according to the mother.
>
> Because the mother reported herself to have emotional problems, and the child's safety was at issue, the child was accepted into temporary voluntary care. The child was placed in a foster home. The foster mother reported that the child had difficulty adjusting. The child was reported not to sleep well,

had constant fits of crying, and did not communicate with the foster mother or other children. The foster mother questioned the child's health or developmental level. An assessment was requested.

Investigation determined that the maternal grandmother was both unwilling and unable to care for the child because of her physical incapacity. She was unwilling because she believed that the mother needed to be more responsible. She further believed that the mother was not sick, that she wanted to be irresponsible and not care for her child. She was willing to assist the agency with information. Contact with the maternal grandmother provided information on the paternal grandmother, who was willing and able to take her grandchild. She believed that children needed to be with family. After less than two weeks in care, the six-year-old was released to the mother, who immediately placed the child in the care of the paternal grandmother. The case was closed with the child's return home.

The Helping Environment

The helping environment is where intervention and prevention occur. The family model for RT/CT (see Figure 8.1) begins with observed behavior. The process of observation includes the observed as well as the observer. The environment is socially constructed and requires involvement. It is the establishment or reestablishment of a warm, intimate, emotional, nurturing environment. Involvement between the practitioner and the family leads to the development of an effective helping relationship. According to Perlman (1979):

> Past those essential physical survival and safety needs that must be assured for every one of us is the need for love, and just past that, perhaps intermingling with it, is our continuous lifelong need for social connectedness, for belonging to and with and for other human beings. Whatever its original ancient adaptive purposes, we seem now to carry in our very genes the need for others. (p. 178)

All constructive efforts toward prevention are based upon this involvement. This provides the psychological environment necessary for change.

The helping environment must, of necessity, focus upon the use of knowledge and values in the prevention process. Our knowledge and values are critical factors in the formation of need-fulfilling pictures and the subsequent behaviors. These are two critical components of the perceptual system. Our perceptions determine our behaviors (Powers, 1973). The family system is composed of processes that provide the foundation upon which practitioners must develop a nurturing environment.

Information input, negative feedback, and the coding process are communicative materials that allow the family to interact with its environment. They are processes that furnish signals to the family about the environment (internal as well as external). They further inform the family about its own functioning and choices in relation to the environment. Coding is the general term for the selective filtering mechanism of a system by which to reject, accept, or translate incoming information for the family. The family, under the auspice of society's ethnic and cultural diversity, selectively filters information to form its own interpretation of the world. Information received from the external environment helps to shape the internal environment. The interpretative process is a function that helps to maintain a sense of balance within the family structure. The therapist must understand, to be effective, the role of selective filtering in interpreting information for the family system. Coding is an important facet in the formation of the quality world.

The filtering process is selective because family systems differ in level and capacity as well as the choices they make in their interaction with the external environment. The perceptual system is composed of filters between the internal world and the external world. These filters are composed of knowledge, values, and our sensory system. Our ability to know the world is based upon what passes through the filters as well as how we choose to interpret it. The filters selectively screen information (energy) from the external world and combine what is left into perceptual reality. Perception is based upon our sensory capacity as well as our knowledge and values.

Coding is the general term for the selective-filtering mechanism of a system by which it rejects, accepts, or translates incoming information. According to Check (1988), "Special senses mediate between the external world and our internal world. These proprio-ceptive senses gather signals from inside the body to provide us with information about where we stand literally—in relation to the external world" (p. 33). Under the auspice of cultural diversity, systems selectively filter their interpretation of the world. It is a function that helps to maintain a sense of balance within their struc-tures. Coding is a two-way interactive process that allows the sys-tem to communicate with its environment. It furnishes signals to a particular system about its environment (internal as well as exter-nal). Morris (1996) states, "Attention is drawn to differences in individual interpretations of situations that can emerge because of differences in gender, class, culture, age group, life experiences, or one's position or role in a group or society" (p. 39). The perceptual system is encoded by families, resulting in a change in behavior. Behavior is the control of perceptions (Powers, 1973).

At times, families fail to communicate effectively (or to have their communication interpreted properly). This does not change their basic needs. The difference is in interpretation of the world and how the needs are communicated. This is crucial to understand-ing the behaviors of families who perceive their world as non-need fulfilling. This has a significant impact upon, and may limit the effectiveness of, prevention or intervention. The family defines its world by what is passed through its filters. The components of the external environment are shaped by gender, class, culture, age, and so on. These are the selective-filtering mechanisms. This filtering results in behaviors that are the family's best attempt to meet its needs in the real world.

Therapists must learn to encode as well as decode the world of those with whom they work. A historical example of the coding process is the slave spiritual. Slaves were able to use their spirituali-ty to reshape religion in the United States and develop the spiritual. Spirituals became songs of religion for the oppressor and songs of freedom for the oppressed. They helped to form a collective con-sciousness among the oppressed that provided hope for a better life in the here and now. The primary focus of the spiritual was commu-nication. This communication was used to enhance identity, protest, rebellion, organization, community collective consciousness, and action. For the oppressed, they were songs of hope for a better life in another world (Mickel, 1995).

The steady state and dynamic homeostasis are concerned with the ratio of energy exchanges and the method whereby relations between parts remain in harmony. The basic principle is the preservation of the character of the family. The family in a homeostasis situation attempts to balance its current functioning with what it perceives as quality living, more commonly termed the "good life." The individual within the family attempts to balance his or her goals with the perceived family goals. The steady state and homeostasis explain how oppressed family structures compensate for their external environment and develop viable functioning systems.

Example: Case Study

When the mother, as a result of her emotional illness, placed her child in temporary care, the family, in its effort to maintain balance, refused to accept illness and chose to define the issue as the mother's irresponsibility. The family chose to view the mother as not fulfilling her responsibility to her child and, therefore, as an irresponsible parent. When confronted with the possibility of placement, the maternal grandmother chose her own illness as rationale for not taking the child. She hoped the mother would keep her own child, and when she did not, the maternal grandmother could explain her own inability to be a resource for the child. These behaviors, whether based on fact or fiction, assisted the family system to maintain a sense of balance—well-being. Due to illness, it became acceptable, temporarily, for a member of the family to be in care. Just as illness allowed the mother to place her child without a sense of failure, illness allowed the maternal grandmother to be unable to assume responsibility. This case illustrates how a family can seek balance through selectively interpreting the world.

African-centered reality therapy addresses the communal nature of intervention and prevention. Basically, our beliefs about families are socially constructed. They develop within the context of our social relationships. Social intervention, of necessity, occurs within a communal context. Within this context, certain procedures lead to change, for example:

> Two individuals who look at the case of a mother who wishes to place her child in temporary foster care can, depending upon knowledge and values, which impact perceptions, come to opposite conclusions: One can choose to view a "dysfunctional family system" and believe placement is in the best interest of the child, with a goal of adoption. Another can choose to expand the vision of the family and see perfectibility and understand polarity—every problem has a solution within it. The family is not limited by blood or frequency of communication and passes the child through the system as quickly as possible and places this child with a "family" member.

The Procedures That Lead to Change

This process continues with an observation of the presenting behavior (see Figure 8.1). Take time to look at what is going on and attempt in your best judgment to determine if this behavior is need fulfilling. The African-centered family practitioner accepts difference as a necessary component in prevention and intervention reality. Difference exists and is an acceptable facet of the reality of the family. Remember that all behavior is an attempt to fulfill some need. Needs are expressed through wants. Always pay particular attention to external behaviors, which are the key to understanding internal needs—yours and the family's. Several questions must be answered when assessing behavior: Is another behavior necessary? Can this behavior be ignored? If not, why not? Answers to these questions usually determine the next step.

The practitioner then moves to ask the client system (family) what it wants. As families move to defining their wants, they become empowered (Solomon, 1976). Empowerment, operationally defined, is helping families take effective control of their lives. Empowered families know in what direction they wish to go. The practitioner who uses empowering practices helps the family to choose the direction intervention will take. The problem-solving process focuses upon what the family wants (see Figure 8.1). It is important to remember that we always plan to the need that will facilitate an understanding of wants and their relationship to basic needs. Once the practitioner understands what the client wants, it then becomes necessary to translate that want into a basic need. This model posits that families cannot always get what they want, but families can always get some of what they need. Determining which need to work on is an important step in the direction toward helping families take effective control of their lives.

Families will take expectations as seriously as the practitioner. The family must take the future in its own hands and engage the transformative process. Families must be prepared to work for the transformation to take place.

Change consists of understanding that the problem is real and that it is time to do something about it. It requires a demonstration of seriousness by doing or not doing (What are you doing? Is it working?—*Stop*) something. Once a decision is made, the next step is to develop a definable, doable plan.

The key components at this point are value judgment, evaluation, and planning. To move to a plan, one must get a value judgment from the family that it wishes to move in a different direction or change behaviors. Family members must make a decision that what they are currently doing either is not working, is against the rules (abusive or neglectful), or is not taking them in the direction they wish to go. Addressing whether behavior is need fulfilling is critical. One must evaluate what is wanted in terms of what is available and realistic. It is also necessary to look at wants in terms of cultural and gender issues.

After an assessment of what is currently being done to get what is wanted, the process moves forward. Once behaviors are assessed, planning can take place. All plans should be success oriented and strength building. They should have built-in milestones and checkpoints. Planning is an ongoing process. The final component of effective planning is commitment. The family must be invested in the plan for it to move forward. It should be remembered that if a plan is to work, there must be a payoff for the family. Therefore, one must make sure it is the family's plan and not the practitioner's. This is easier said than done. It is always necessary to include a commitment within any success-oriented plan. Finally, the plan must also be evaluated to determine if it is indeed working.

The foundation of this perspective is the knowledge and value system that is essential for making a shift to an African-centered paradigm. This paradigm is especially useful for those working with African-American families. New paradigms transform our perception of both the form and function of the family system. That transformation begins with a review of our epistemology and axiology models. Forward-looking thinkers must establish an African-American philosophy to govern what happens to families. When one works with the family, he or she must use a paradigm that appreciates the struggle to overcome oppression. It must further be recognized that what is good for African-American families will be good for all families. The African-centered paradigm provides a foundation for restructuring prevention and intervention.

CONCLUSION

When one works with the African-American family, he or she must use a frame of reference that appreciates the struggle for empowerment. When using this perspective, one receives a sense that although there may be problems, solutions are near. Those who would promote hopelessness and failure are not in tune with the principles that uplift. All relationships work, and those which seem to be less than perfect contain perfection. The family has the wherewithal to move from a non-need-fulfilling position to another stage of development. It is at this stage that one uses the principles that demonstrate a culturally competent perspective and thereby enhance the need-fulfilling relationship. The principle must also support the traditional values of the African-American family. These values are important to the African-American community but may be at odds with those who perceive this community as valueless. It is therefore important that the practitioner deals with the reality of external and internal environments. To be most effective, the practitioner must choose the appropriate time for intervention and prevention. Each family has a rhythm. The practitioner must evaluate that rhythm and determine when the family is ready to engage in the helping process. For example, consider the voluntary placement of a child:

The most appropriate time for intervention was after the child had been placed in a foster home. The family's vision was that all children belonged at home (with a family member). Placement unbalanced this family and its perception of quality child rearing. Family members were, at this point, willing and able, once the child was placed, to help identify a family resource. Prior to placement, intervention was inappropriate for the rhythm of the family.

There are periods of readiness, and the practitioner must be in tune with this environment to intervene at the appropriate time. When the system is ready to receive information and act on it, families can restructure. There is always a time and a way to make change. It is imperative that the practitioner move to bring about change when the family is ready. If the atmosphere within the family is not appropriate, change will be rejected. Families develop in time, in concert with communities, where they are free to choose the time of change.

Timing is concerned with when and where change occurs. An assessment of the family, based on locating the strengths and reinforcing the areas of need, is conducive to change if that change is introduced in the right way at the right time. In any event, a change in one part brings about concomitant changes in all parts. This is a basic tenet of all social systems. The analysis can determine when and where maximal intervention occurs.

The method is to analyze the whole, and from this analysis, we are able to utilize the union of opposites. The African-centered approach to work with the family seems to be the method of choice. The family and its members are, in the final analysis, the only viable change agents. Thus, what is proposed here is a way to involve the family in an empowering change process that will responsibly meet its needs.

What are your expectations from what you do as an intervener? Do you believe in and have you developed a commitment to empowerment? Pathology is an aberration; it is not expected—wellness is. Conservation of the past is essential to understanding our oneness. No matter how well a structure is built it must stand on something. A people's history is a people's memory, and memory is the bridge that carries families over troubled moments. Recommitment to our highest ideals, the human personality, and the African-centered matrix provide the foundation for a self-fulfilling prophecy. The self-fulfilling prophecy posits that African-centered prevention and intervention under reality therapy/choice theory is a viable alternative for those who wish to consider a different way to work with families.

REFERENCES

Ani, M. (1994). *Yurugu.* Trenton, NJ: Africa World Press, Inc.
Asante, M.K. (1988). *Afrocentricity.* Trenton, NJ: Africa World Press, Inc.
Asante, M.K. and Asante, K.W. (Eds.) (1990). *African culture: The rhythms of unity.* Trenton, NJ: Africa World Press, Inc.
Azibo, D.A. (1989). African-centered theses on mental health and a nosology of black/African personality disorder. *The Journal of Black Psychology, 15*(2), 173-214.
Baldwin, J.A. (1986). African (black) psychology: Issues and synthesis. *Journal of Black Studies, 16*(2), 235-249.
Beckett, J.O. and Johnson, H.C. (1995). Human development. In R.L. Edwards and J.G. Hopps (Eds.), *Encyclopedia of social work* (pp. 1385-1405). Washington, DC: NASW.
Budge, E.A. (1960). *The book of the dead.* New Hyde Park, NY: University Books, Inc.
Canda, E. (1988). Spirituality, religious diversity, and social work practice. *Social Casework, 69*(2), 238-247.
Carruthers, J. (1980). Reflections on the history of the Afrocentric worldview. *Black Books Bulletin, 7*(11), 4-7, 13, 25.
Check, W.A. (1988). *Drugs and perception.* New York: Chelsea House.
Cornett, C. (1992). Toward a more comprehensive personology: Integrating a spiritual perspective into social work practice. *Social Work, 37*(2), 101-102.
Fanon, F. (1967). *Black skin, white masks.* New York: Grove Press.
Glasser, W. (1965). *Reality therapy.* New York: Harper & Row.
Glasser, W. (1980). *What are you doing?* New York: Harper & Row.
Glasser, W. (1988). Dr. Glasser's corner. *William Glasser Institute Newsletter, 3,* Summer. Conoga Park, CA: Institute for Reality Therapy.
Glasser, W. (1996). *A message from Dr. William Glasser.* May 22, 1996.
Glasser, W. (1998). *Choice theory.* New York: HarperCollins.
Institute for Reality Therapy (1987). *Policies and procedures manual.* Los Angeles: Author.
Joseph, G.G., Reddy, V., and Searle-Chatterjee, M. (1990). Eurocentrism in the social sciences. *Race and Class, 31*(4), 1-24.
Karenga, M. (1984). *Selections from the Husia.* Los Angeles: Kawaida Publications.

Karenga, M. (1989). *The African American holiday of Kwanzaa.* Los Angeles: University of Sankore Press.

Karenga, M. (1990). *The book of coming forth by day.* Los Angeles: University of Sankore Press.

Massey, G. (1970). *Ancient Egypt.* New York: Samuel Weiser.

Mbiti, J.S. (1969). *African religions and philosophy.* London: Heinemann.

Mickel, E. (1990). Family therapy utilizing control theory: A systems perspective. *Journal of Reality Therapy, 10*(1), 26-33.

Mickel, E. (1991). Integrating the African centered perspective with reality therapy/control theory. *Journal of Reality Therapy, 11*(1), 66-71.

Mickel, E. (1993). Parent Assistance Workshops (P.A.W.S.) reality based intervention for the crack exposed child. *Journal of Reality Therapy, 12*(2), 20-28.

Mickel, E. (1995). *The black church and self help: Spirituals and spirituality.* Paper presented at the 13th Annual Baccalaureate Program Director Conference, Nashville, Tennessee, October 26-29.

Minnich, E.K. (1990). *Transforming knowledge.* Philadelphia: Temple University Press.

Morris, T. (1996). The struggle to recognize everyday social work as rational practice. *Arete, 20*(2), 36-41.

Perlman, H. (1979). *Relationship: The heart of helping people.* Chicago: The University of Chicago Press.

Powers, W. (1973). *Behavior: The control of perception.* Chicago: Aldine Publishing Company.

Richards, D. (1990). The implications of African-American spirituality. In M.K. Asante and K.W. Asante (Eds.), *African culture: The rhythms of unity* (pp. 207-231). Trenton, NJ: Africa World Press, Inc.

Semmes, C.E. (1981). Foundations of an Afrocentric social science: Implications for curriculum-building, theory, and research in black studies. *Journal of Black Studies, 12*(1), 3-17.

Solomon, B. (1976). *Black empowerment: Social work in oppressed communities.* New York: Columbia University Press.

Somé, M.P. (1993). *Of water and the spirit.* New York: G.P. Putnam's Sons.

Thompson, J.D. (1967). *Organizations in action.* New York: McGraw-Hill.

Three Initiates (1988). *The Kybalion.* Clayton, GA: Tri-State Press.

Chapter 9

Reclaiming the Inner Strength: An Expanded Perspective for Working with Inner-City Families

Sadye L. Logan

The overall quality of life in the United States has been affected by the escalation of violence and other risk conditions. Although no segment of American society can escape this condition, the impact is most often felt in the inner cities or urban areas, where the majority of the residents are poor families and children of color. Here, the concentration of poverty and segregation gives rise to a social context of drug use, welfare dependency, teenage parenthood, and violence as the norm. In addition to a nonnurturing family life, most young people growing up in urban areas also experience poor-quality education and strong peer pressures not to succeed in school or to drop out and adopt an attitude of "getting over" (an expression suggesting that a person has not earned what they have). Such learned behavior is viewed as counterproductive to building and sustaining hopefulness (Ogbu and Fordham, 1986).

Several authors have suggested that to create expectations of hope for inner-city families and to move them out of the poverty trap requires an expanded approach to helping (Logan, 1996; Schiele, 1996). Therefore, this chapter proposes an expanded perspective for working with inner-city families. It describes a contextually based approach for addressing family dynamics, in terms of structure and functions. Such an approach refers to the biopsychosocial, spiritual, and historical factors that impact upon the family's life and is conceptualized in terms of life domains (see Table 9.1):

recreation/socialization, self-image, guidance, family cooperation, health (mental and physical), and economics. These domains are discussed in more detail later in the chapter. This chapter also provides specific and mutual helping strategies for fostering hope and positive change within families.

TABLE 9.1. The Family Functioning Continuum

Life Domains	Stable: Nurturing or Functioning Well	Less Stable: Midrange Functioning	Severely Unstable: Dysfunctional or Nonnurturing
Recreation/ Socialization	People feel loving. People feel free to talk about inside feelings. All feelings are okay and members can play together. Strong parental coalition.	People have difficulty putting feelings into words. Most feelings are okay and can be talked about. Children are sometimes triangulated by a parent.	Hurt and disappointment are typical reactions in the family. People compulsively protect inside feelings. Only "certain" feelings are okay. Coalitions exist across generations.
Self-image	Individual differences are accepted. Members are considered more important than performance. Each member likes self and respects others. People have high self-worth.	Some conformity is encouraged. Some ambivalence re: person versus performance. Most times individuals like selves and are respectful of others. People's self-worth fluctuates.	Everyone must conform to strongest person's ideas, values. Performance is considered more important than the person. People have low self-worth.
Guidance	Each person responsible for own actions. Respectful criticisms and appropriate consequences for actions. There are very few shoulds for other members.	Some control over action of others. Sometimes guilt is activated as the consequence for actions. There are some shoulds for other members. Rules are sometimes ambiguous.	Lots of control, criticism. Punishment and shaming are typically used as consequences. Lots of shoulds for members. Unclear, inconsistent, and rigid rules.

Family Cooperation	People are planful. Decisions are shared. Roles are easily reversed and shared. People compromise easily.	People are usually planful. Decisions are often shared. Roles are somewhat flexible. People compromise.	Everything is spur-of-the-moment. Decisions are not shared. Roles are rigidly defined. People do not compromise.
Health (Mental and Physical)	All subjects open to discussion. Atmosphere is relaxed and joyous. The system faces and works through stress. People have energy. Growth is celebrated.	Some subjects are not open to discussion. Atmosphere sometimes tense and stressful. People are usually energetic. Growth is discouraged in most areas.	There are many taboo subjects, lots of secrets. Atmosphere is tense. Lots of anger, fear. The system avoids stress. People feel tired. Growth is threatening and thus discouraged.
Economics	People feel financially secure. People are gainfully employed. There is support for training or studying for job promotion or change in careers. Adequate living arrangements.	People are financially solvent. People are employed or in training programs. Living arrangements may be crowded, but adequate.	People feel financially insecure. People are not gainfully employed. No thoughts of training or study for job promotion or career change. Inadequate living arrangements.

Source: Adapted from Logan, Freeman, and McRoy, 1990, pp. 78-79.

PHILOSOPHICAL AND PRACTICE EXPERIENCES

In part, helping families to connect with their inner strengths, sometimes referred to as holistic healing, has evolved out of the author's long practice and research experience with families and children, especially families and children of color. A complementary experience emerged from a year-long sabbatical that was spent in residence at the Child Guidance and Family Therapy Training Center in Philadelphia. The sabbatical experience served to corroborate perceptions about the magnitude of issues and concerns confronting inner-city families of color, but it also affirmed the need for developing more holistic ways of thinking about and responding to the needs of troubled families and children living in the inner cities.

Although the experience at the Family Therapy Training Center was enriched by a network of affiliated services from a major hospital, a medical school, a psychiatric and pediatric department, and a diverse grouping of programs and services, something less tangible was missing. This missing link was partially captured in the center's view and utilization of ecological systems as a natural and essential resource in the helping/healing process. For example, ecological systems thinking focuses on the assumptions that systems are mutually interacting and that the nature of this interaction provides basic information about how problems come into existence and are sustained, the nature of interaction and behavior, and the course of human development (Compton and Galaway, 1999). It would follow that if these mutually interacting systems provide information about how problems are developed and sustained, then they should also provide information about how problems might be resolved. A practice example that utilizes ecological systems conceptualization is reflected in a special agency's project focusing on grandparent-headed families (Buchanan and Lappin, 1990). The project leaders were severely challenged by the families and the concerns that they brought to the project. Grandmothers were the primary caretakers of the families being served. According to Buchanan and Lappin (1990, p. 49), these families had *"been robbed of the very soul of their identities as families"* (italics added).

Many of the families, although not grandparent-headed, fit this category also. However, the most amazing thing about these families is that they are not completely devoid of hope. The souls of their identities as families and as individuals may have been severely damaged, but somehow they have faith in the institutionalized image of hope that the center represented for inner-city families. These families were some of the most difficult treatment cases, and many were eventually lost through the cracks of the helping process. More must be done for these families as well as all inner-city families. In addition to rewriting treatment texts, we must also expand our vision and beliefs in people, in the abilities and strengths of the less fortunate in this society.

HOLISTIC HEALING
AS A THEORETICAL CONSTRUCT

Overview

In some ways, this proposed perspective is grounded in the visionary work of scholars such as Bertha Reynolds (1975) and Ruth Smalley (1958). Currently, this perspective is referred to as mind/body work and involves approaches to healing or helping that include meditation, massage, guided imagery, herbal prescriptions, acupuncture, and biofeedback. However, at a more basic level, the perspective refers to healing communities that are concerned with the strengths of families and the community in which they live. The focus is on bringing all aspects of being together to support the healing process. Within this context, healing communities are pivotal in addressing needs and concerns holistically (Smith, 1993). In addressing the whole human being, attention is focused on the physical, emotional, social, and spiritual. These components are viewed as interrelated and therefore must be addressed as an integrated whole. A critical factor in this process is the powerful impact of the mind on the body (Gillett, 1992). The emerging body of literature and research in this area seems to be in agreement that both the person providing the service and the recipient of the service must assume more expanded roles for effective mind/body work (Lerner, 1993; Remen, 1993; Kabat-Zinn, 1993). However, to operationalize the notion that each one is responsible for one's own healing, and has the capability to do so, requires a shift in our thinking and ways of doing.

As suggested earlier, an essential factor in this expanded or new paradigm of helping is the recognition of the power of the mind in determining our life course (Swami Anantananda, 1996; Felton, 1993; Gillett, 1992). Kabat-Zinn (1993) suggests that the goal in mind/body work is to help people face their issues and concerns, to notice the mind's reactions, and to let go of that reactivity. He goes on to say that with practice and consistency, one can come to find an inner stillness and peace within some of the most difficult situations. In this process, people come to learn how to step back from their thought processes and recognize that they are not their thoughts, but the ones who are observing the thoughts. This is empowerment. As people learn more and more how to watch their thoughts, they can decide which to pay attention to and which to ignore. In this way, people begin to live more fully from moment to moment, with a greater sense of control over their lives.

Earlier helpers recognized the potential of putting clients in charge of their lives and building on existing strengths as a means to release inner resources (Reynolds, 1975; Smalley, 1953, 1958). Current trends suggest the importance of continuing in the tradition of Bertha Reynolds and others to activate internal healing processes. This movement rests on the belief that people have inherent inner strengths and are able to grow and develop when this strength is tapped and affirmed (Logan, 1994; Saleebey, 1992). Further, it appears, in some ways, that the healing process and the helping process are being conceptualized interchangeably (Bass and Davis, 1988; Calvi, 1988; Levine, 1987). With a view toward using the concepts interchangeably, this chapter defines the healing process, on one level, as professional helpers helping others to help themselves—put another way, professionals empowering or supporting others on their journey back to health. Overall, this view of helping is central to this conceptualization of inner healing and is supported by the branch of medicine called "psychosomatic medicine." Psychosomatic medicine explores the mind-body connection and purports that when one is happy and centered, the body has greater resistance to illness. Likewise, when one is anxious or depressed, many more physical illnesses are likely to occur (Felton, 1993). Implicit in this view of healing is the powerful influence of the mind on the body. This suggests the need to better understand the epistemology of the mind as well as to practice being "centered" in the body for more balance and a healthy life.

Centering As a Healing Concept

It follows that an essential component of holistic healing is centering, a process that may be viewed as connected to all aspects of functioning. It is a process that suggests that people must be valued and affirmed. It builds on the notion that all human beings, including those needing professional help with problems in living, possess a wealth of untapped internal and external resources that sometimes manifest externally in the form of talents, dreams, aspirations, hope, and myriad other unconscious or subconscious strengths. It is the wellspring of inner strengths that is often overlooked or neglected by clients and their helpers. To begin the process of activating one's awareness of these strengths, it is useful to begin with the following set of assumptions about human beings:

1. An inherent inner strength or life force exists within each human being. This inner strength is the essence of who we are and directs our growth and development (Swami Chidvilasananda, 1989; Logan, 1994; Saleebey, 1992).
2. When people are affirmed and adopt a positive mind-set about their worth and value as human beings, an inner and outer transformation occurs (Logan, 1994; Reynolds, 1975).
3. Empowerment is a process that must be moved from outside to inside (to be owned by the person) for permanent healing to occur (Lee, 1994; Solomon, 1976).
4. Problems should be viewed as friends/teachings about life that bring about personal growth and help in finding solutions to life issues (Furman and Ahola, 1992).

Unfortunately, most people, especially those in need of professional help, have great difficulty becoming firmly established in their own center or even accepting some of the previous assumptions about themselves. Why is this? Is it because most people do not know what constitutes their essential nature or know where their centers are (see Covey, 1989)? This lack of centering is directly related to one's difficulty in remaining connected to one's own feelings. Although this condition is true for most people, it is especially true for troubled families and children. The families and children of the inner cities are especially vulnerable to numerous problems in living, such as racism, and many social deprivations that mitigate against being centered. These problems create stress that permeates their lives and keeps them perpetually other focused, that is, focused on blaming, self-hate, and many self-defeating patterns of behavior. These problems in living often manifest for these families in the form of violence, substance abuse, chronic and acute illnesses, and cripplingly low self-esteem. These external circumstances, and numerous other powerful forces, tend to freeze families' ways of being and thinking at a very basic level of functioning.

When this process occurs, people become dysfunctional or ineffectual in day-to-day living (Calvi, 1988; Remen, 1993).

Figure 9.1 captures the dynamic of the centering process as well as the process for changing it. The figure suggests in the first circle that most people's awareness of their existence is externally based. In other words, outside conditions and situations or other people's attitudes determine one's feelings and reactions to life events. The second circle focuses on the self of the person. Self-awareness is a concept that suggests that many people habitually feel bad or cultivate some negative state of being. For many people, feeling bad or negative seems to be a natural condition. Although they wish to cultivate a different feeling, they go on doing more of the same (see Swami Anantananda, 1996; Gillett, 1992). In addition, as already suggested, Figure 9.1 not only reflects the process but the conditions for changing this negative mind-set. At the innermost circle, pure awareness, or one's state of being, exists with the potential for freeing one from problems in living. Being centered in this awareness, one comes to see that many of the feelings being experienced are habitual and need not be that way simply because it appears to have always been that way (Swami Anantananda, 1996). It is an affirmation that something outside or someone else does not have the power to make one feel bad against one's will or against one's choosing. Calvi (1988) describes this process as laying down the weapons around the heart. These weapons are anything that keeps one from experiencing life fully.

The Means of Accomplishing Centering

Building on Figure 9.1, Figure 9.2 reflects the "cause" as well as the "cure" for the quality of one's existence that brings joyful or painful experience. The diagram suggests that when one loses *hope,* it is due to *scarcity* in some form—a condition that results in feelings of *hopelessness.* The same order of reasoning follows the other four (commitment/greed, faith/violence) conditions. One's beliefs about these conditions and their impact upon oneself determines one's experience of being in the world. Another way of expressing this is that people cannot always determine what will happen to them, but they can always determine what happens *in* them by controlling what they *think* (Borysenko, 1988; Gillett, 1992). For

FIGURE 9.1. The Centering Process

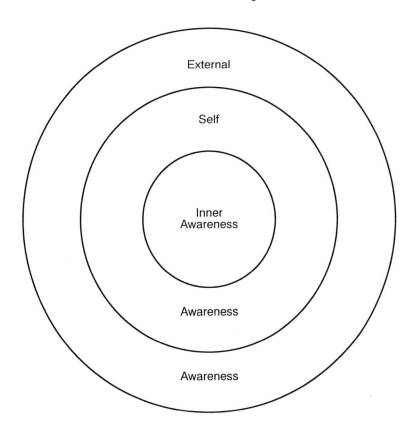

Goal: To change the script of one's life.

example, you have worked very hard for a promotion and your superior hints of a positive outcome, but the promotion is denied. You cannot prevent your superior from denying the promotion, but you can determine your experience of this outcome, simply through controlling what you think about it—in essence, staying centered in your inner being.

FIGURE 9.2. The Human Condition

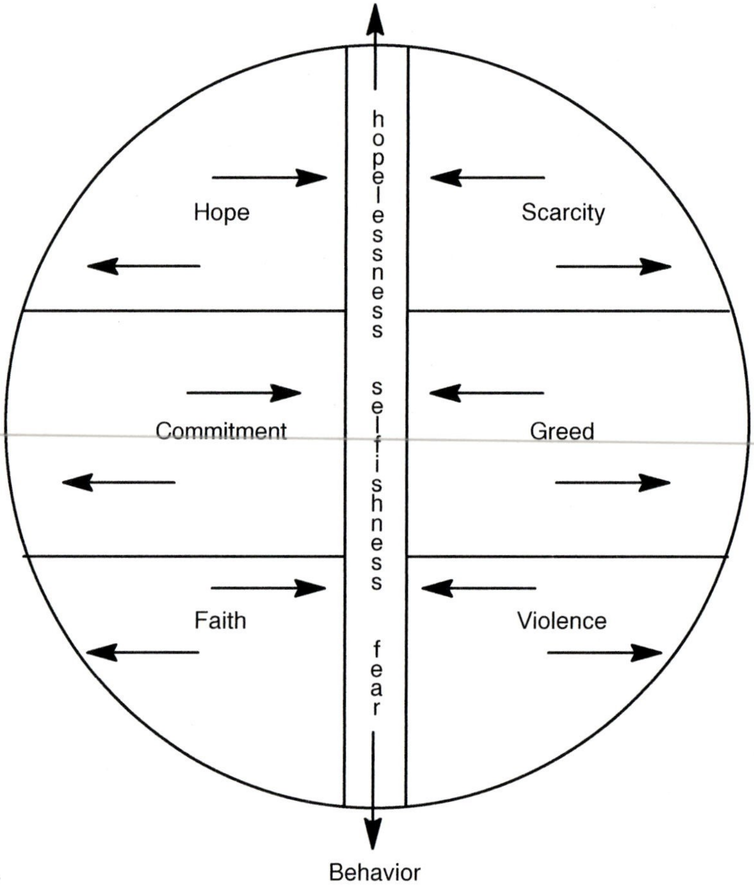

Applying this level of reasoning and analysis to family dynamics and functioning suggests that families must change their life scripts or stories of living/being in the world to change their lives (Coles, 1984; White and Epston, 1990). Of course, this is not an easy process, but it is not an impossible task either. To some extent, the work with families to bring about such changes is already being done in a variety of contexts, but it must evolve beyond special situations (Buchanan and Lappin, 1990; Remen, 1993; Smith, 1993) and become a part of our ongoing practice repertoire. For this to happen, professional helpers and educators must become more vigilant and more committed to understanding this expanded view of helping.

The remaining discussion on principles of holistic practice will address ways to operationalize this perspective and practical strategies for helping families to reclaim their inner strengths.

The Principles of Holistic Practice

The holistic principles of practice build upon existing practice principles and are based on the four assumptions previously addressed. Together these factors serve as a framework for operationalizing these principles. Four principles of holistic practice are connected with this approach. These principles are not new but are presented in an expanded context. Included are (1) joining, (2) building understanding and recognizing strengths, (3) identifying goals, and (4) building expectations.

The First Principle: Joining with the Family

Effective joining is critical. Generally, by the time inner-city families seek professional intervention they have exhausted personal attempts at solving the presenting concern. At this stage in the helping encounter, it is important to demonstrate respect and concern for the family and to do everything possible to reduce unnecessary obstacles to a trusting, open communication.

The Second Principle: Exploring the Family's Understanding of, and Interaction with, Their Environment

Table 9.1 is useful in this process. The six life domains frame this search for strengths that sustain and support the family. The life domains are as follows.

Recreation/socialization, the first life domain, focuses on the nature and quality of the family's emotional and social supports: What do family members do for fun, individually, or as a unit? How are children viewed, parented, and integrated into the family functioning?

Self-image, the second domain, examines the family's perceptions about self and others: To what extent were dreams deferred? How does the family view itself racially or ethnically?

Guidance, the third domain, is concerned with the family's values, attitudes, beliefs, rituals, and myths. This domain also explores the family's religious and spiritual orientation: What is the family's coping philosophy? Is the church and/or other spiritual/cultural organization relied on as an important resource?

Family cooperation, the fourth domain, addresses the family vocation and chores and allows for the exploration of role conflict, role confusion, role reversal, and role overload: Who does the family depend on for support? To what extent is role sharing practiced?

Health (physical and mental), the fifth domain, explores an often neglected area of functioning. This domain reflects the family's ability to maintain a balance between inner needs and outer demands (staying centered) in carrying out daily tasks. It is also concerned with the family's response to health care: What are the family's cultural beliefs and patterns regarding health issues? Is the family generally flexible, in touch with feelings, motivated, and able to follow through?

Economics, the sixth and final domain, explores the family's living arrangements and financial resources. Here, the focus is on the family's level of satisfaction with the physical setting of home and neighborhood, family members' values and attitudes concerning their financial status, and how they choose to and would like to use their income: What resources are available and not being utilized? What are the least and greatest things that would raise the level of satisfaction with home, the neighborhood, and financial resources?

The majority of the families living in the inner cities fall between the less stable and severely unstable end of the continuum. The family discussed later in this chapter fits this category. However, the children's experiences are best described as severely unstable until committed to live with their grandmother.

The Third Principle: Identifying Concrete, Measurable, Achievable Goals That Empower the Family

The exploration of needs and identifying goals are based on the presenting concerns. The focus is on what the family wants to change and what in the past stopped change from occurring. The specific tasks to be accomplished are determined by the family's capacity, motivation, and opportunities. This means that work should be incremental and at the family's pace. In other words, *go slow.*

The Fourth Principle: The Creation of Hope or Expectation

The first of several strategies identified with achieving hope deals with helping family members to separate themselves or their attitudes from the presenting concerns. Some authors refer to this process as externalizing the problem (Epston, 1994; White and Epston, 1990). It is viewed as a way of helping clients to move out of the world of problems into the world of experiences, new possibilities, and new opportunities. This task is achieved by helping family members map the influence of the presenting concern in their lives and relationships as well as to map the influence of the family in the life of the problem: What one thing or occasion did the family not allow the problem to control?

In addition to creating expectations through the search for exceptions (De Shazer et al., 1986), the following strategies strengthen, promote inner strengths, and activate the healing process:

1. The first strategy concerns the utilization of the "seven healing sayings":

- "I am loved" or "I love you"
- "I am grateful" or "Thank you"
- "I care" or "I am sorry"
- "I do not know" or "I need help"
- "I expect more" or "That's not good enough"
- "Everything happens for the best" or "Nothing happens by chance"
- "I have had enough and will not take anymore" or "No! Stop! Enough!"

Other practitioners and authors have used similar expressions to convey a movement toward activating the inner strengths and ownership of present situations and life in general. Not unlike Calvi's

(1988) expressions of encouragement, these expressions help clients determine the fullness of their emotional and spiritual lives. In other words, they are a useful way of checking level of centeredness. Clients are instructed to ask themselves, "Which of these seven messages are the easiest to say? The most frequently uttered? Which are the most difficult to say? Are there some which are never uttered? Does the pattern remain constant regardless of who you are with—family, co-workers, friends?" Each of the sayings expresses feelings or a state that fosters growth, empowerment, and inner transformation. Absence of any one denotes a degree of spiritual starvation or "dryness" of the heart.

"I love you" or "I am loved" as an unconditional expression of caring and respect is the most expansive of the seven messages. It releases all of one's natural emotions—joy, bliss, contentment, trust, peace. "Thank you" or an expression of gratitude is an acknowledgment of our interconnectedness, of receiving and appreciating. Although this is an extremely difficult expression for people who have been oppressed or the recipient of numerous injustices or abuses, it is a necessary and critical movement toward centeredness. "I am sorry" or "I care" is a powerful expression of humility. It also demonstrates that humility is not an expression of weakness, but one of strength. "I need help" or "I do not know" is a message based on the conviction that one's emotional and spiritual needs will be or are being met and that one feels secure. However, many are reluctant to send this message, based on their beliefs or understanding about the source or origin of true helping. Also connected to the reluctance are feelings of unworthiness about receiving help. "I expect more" or "That's not good enough" is a powerful message of hopefulness. It expresses self-worth, self-esteem, and self-love. "I have had enough and will not take anymore" or "No! Stop! Enough!" is a message about establishing boundaries and appropriately connecting with the power of anger and indignation. Together, these seven strengths-based expressions create a foundation for continued growth and healing.

2. The second strategy involves teaching families to *respond* instead of *reacting* to life circumstances. For example, to help the grandmother who is described in the following case illustration to practice listening more and talking less, to search for alternative

responses to yelling or some punitive disciplinary measures. This strategy teaches families to separate the emotional part of their functioning from the rational or intellectual part and to have some choice about the degree to which each type of functioning governs their behavior (Kerr and Bowen, 1988).

3. The third strategy teaches families to restory their lives by changing those aspects of their current life scripts that are not working. The centering process serves as the vehicle for initiating this change. This process will allow the mind and body to act out and live the new story. As family members practice living their lives in the way they would like them to be, their lives will change. Again, for the grandmother and her grandchildren, this restorying begins with the recognition that the children's natural parents are sick and may not be able to reassume care and responsibility for them. The life circumstances of the parents need to be placed in perspective, and the children and the grandmother affirmed to allow inner healing to occur.

4. The fourth strategy deals with issues concerning transitioning and new adjustments. Here, families are cautioned that change takes time but that healing is under their control, as the source of the healing power rests within them.

A Case Illustration

Louise, a sixty-five-year-old African-American grandmother from Buchanan and Lappin's (1990) grandparent project will be the case study used for further discussion of the holistic practice principles. This case was selected because it vividly captures the raw struggles of life in the inner city. The case is also representative of families from the author's practice as well as from the practicum caseloads of the author's students.

> Louise is the caretaker and guardian of three grandchildren: Janet, fourteen; Derek, twelve; and Krista, two and a half. Derek is the person targeted as the one with the problem. Derek is described as a sullen, angry boy who has been held back once in school and appears to be failing again. His teachers are fed up with his mouthy attitude and clownish horseplay. The school counselor has talked with Louise several

times. Louise quietly listened to the standard discipline-begins-at-home lecture, not even bothering to voice her real feeling that, "When he's in school, he's your problem." Derek's mother, Sheila, is a crack addict, and his father is in jail for drug dealing.

Prior to the children moving in with their grandmother, they lived with their mother, whose crack addiction made her totally dysfunctional. She ceased functioning as a parent to the point of selling the family's food to support her addiction. Janet and Derek were truant from school for most of the year. Janet had become sexually active and acquired a sexually transmitted disease by her twelfth birthday. Janet's cheerful disposition and strong capacity for survival allowed her to cope with her mother's exaggerated mood swings and avoid physical abuse. Derek, on the other hand, suffered from constant physical abuse by his mother. A sideways glance or a barely audible mutter earned him a scar from a fist, belt buckle, or electric iron cord. Derek became a runner and began sleeping in abandoned cars. With the birth of Sheila's crack-addicted and neurologically impaired baby girl, Krista, Louise recognized the magnitude of her daughter's and her grandchildren's problems. Louise, the hospital, and Child Protective Services intervened. Louise reluctantly became a full-time mother again.

Parenting troubled adolescent grandchildren at age sixty-five is no small task. In addition to being ambivalent about taking on the parenting role, Louise was distrustful of professional helpers.

To analyze this case within the context of the previously discussed holistic principles, it would be useful to view the principles in two parts: The first part includes the first, second, and third principles. These principles establish the context for work. The work begins with recognition and understanding of the complexity of the situation. This includes the grandmother's reluctance, effective joining, affirmation and acknowledgment of strengths, and the search for exceptions through assessing the life domains. These are important and necessary factors in empowering and supporting the grandmother in her parenting role. Part two builds on part one to move the family members individually and collectively toward change and growth. The focus is on demanding concrete, specific tasks from families. It supports the healing process by encouraging families such as Louise's to interact in ways that are affirming and growth enhancing. For example, practice the language of caring: tracking the number, times, and different ways to express the seven healing sayings.

Situations similar to Louise's not only require new and expanded treatment strategies such as those previously discussed, but also requires professional helpers with expanded visions. This expanded vision begins with the five practice assumptions stated earlier, in addition to the following beliefs or assumptions about the inherent worth and resiliency of human beings:

1. People will change because change is inevitable (Swami Chidvilasananda, 1989; Watzlawick, Weakland, and Fisch, 1974).
2. People are naturally seekers and creators of their own realities (Swami Chidvilasananda, 1989; Furman and Ahola, 1992).
3. People have predominant ways of being and responding to events in this world (Swami Chidvilasananda, 1989).
4. People have the capacity to heal themselves or change the conditions of their lives that are causing pain in some form (Swami Chidvilasananda, 1989; Levine, 1987).

The Role of the Practitioner

Implicit in these assumptions is the belief that helpers are merely compassionate guides in the process of helping families to reclaim their strength and to heal themselves. They are "invited" by those in pain to assist them on their journey back to health. They must never own the family issues. In the previous case, the helper realized through the support of the treatment team that Louise did not need to be "fixed" but to grow into wholeness through the support, compassion, and respect she provided. This does not mean to suggest, however, that helpers sit behind a desk and wait for an invitation to offer help. This perspective is, in large part, an internal posture assumed by the worker. Assuming a compassionate stance in helping requires ongoing self-inquiry and reflective thinking regarding one's values, beliefs, and attitudes and their impact on families. It is also imperative to assess the impact of privilege and power in the life of the client and the helper. The external response is based on the impact of these factors and individualizing the client's need. Initially, this may mean home and school visits, creating or working with existing community resources, and providing maximum support with day-to-day living. Buchanan and Lappin (1990) spoke of this awareness on the part of the worker as listening to the grandmother closely, without trying to persuade her of anything. In this way, the worker was able to appreciate the oppressive sense of isolation that dominates the grandmother's life and her disappointment at Derek's rejection of her attempt to help him. It is at this point that the worker might also begin the search for exceptions to the family's concerns: When does the problem not occur, or when is it less? If, in the future, the problem is being solved or has lessened, what are you/others doing differently when it is solved or lessened? It has been demonstrated that exceptions to problems contain hope, faith, abilities, resources, and clues to solutions. In other words, the push is to help families tap into their inherent strengths.

When people are severely scarred emotionally and spiritually, much front-end or supportive work is necessary to assist them in activating the healing process. The supportive work was begun with Louise and her grandchildren. However, helpers must always remember that for long-term change to occur, families that are experiencing the pain must eventually own this work and cultivate hope through the daily practices of the healing messages and their new script for living together as a family. This new script continues to evolve out of the utilization of the five basic strategies and the seven healing assumptions.

Practice Effectiveness

Essentially, this approach to helping focuses on assisting families to access their deep inner resources or strengths for healing, modifying the destructive thought patterns of the mind, and living more effectively in the world. In many ways, this orientation to helping is not new. However, the focus on accessing and reclaiming deep inner strengths as a form of treatment intervention is new. Further, it is an approach that may be viewed by many helping professionals as not the thing to do, at least not immediately. In part, this response is connected to the nature of the intervention that is based on internal individualized experiences. In addition, measuring the effects of what the interventions intended to achieve is an extremely complex matter. Kabat-Zinn (1993) suggests that we have decades worth of studies to do to begin to articulate what it means to go into deep states of relaxation and to change one's relationship to one's own body in terms of the actual felt experiences of it. Another part of this challenge is to work toward helping others to change their way of thinking about and experiencing the world in which they live.

Despite evidence that suggests a positive impact of several types of alternative interventions (prayer, meditation, relaxation techniques), the National Research Council and other dissenters severely criticize these approaches (see Canda, 1998; Dossey, 1993). It is important, however, that helpers work to create an evaluative context for studying the social, psychological, cognitive, and spiritual impact of alternative intervention strategies on clients' overall functioning and well-being.

CONCLUSION

It is becoming increasingly evident that effective helping for troubled families must be directed to the rekindling of faith, hope, meaning, direction, and purpose. This is an ongoing process and, for many, a lifelong process. In this regard, professional helpers must assume expanded perspectives of helping. This style of practice relies on flexibility and the helper's ability to encourage the use of different truths and realities. These perspectives must not only include current practice wisdoms but also be rooted in a postmodern paradigm. In other words, helpers must assume a respectful stance that not only supports and honors families' strengths but is collaborative and builds expectations for change.

REFERENCES

Bass, E. and Davis, L. (1988). *The courage to heal: A guide for women survivors of child sexual abuse.* New York: Harper & Row.
Borysenko, J. (1988). *Minding the body, mending the mind.* New York: Bantam.

Buchanan, B. and Lappin, J. (1990). Restoring the soul of the family: Grandparent-headed families fight the odds against survival. *The Family Therapy Networks, 14*(6) (November/December), 48-52.

Calvi, J. (May 1988). Six healing sayings. *Friends Journal,* 18-19.

Canda, E. (1998). *Spirituality and social work.* Binghamton, NY: The Haworth Press, Inc.

Coles, R. (1984). *The call of stories.* Boston: Houghton Mifflin Company.

Compton, B. and Galaway, B. (1999). *Social work processes.* Pacific Grove, CA: Brooks/Cole Publishing Company.

Covey, S.R. (1989). *The seven habits of highly effective people: Restoring the character ethic.* New York: Simon and Schuster.

De Shazer, S., Berg, I.K., Lipchik, E., Nunally, E., Molnar, A., Gingerich, W., and Weiner-Davis, M. (1986). Brief therapy: Focused solution development. *Family Process, 25,* 207-222.

Dossey, L. (1993). *Healing words.* San Francisco: Harper.

Epston, D. (1994). Extending the conversation. *The Family Networker, 18*(6), 30-37, 62-63.

Felton, D. (1993). The brain and the immune system. In Bill Moyers (Ed.), *Healing and the mind* (pp. 213-237). New York: Doubleday.

Furman, B. and Ahola, T. (1992). *Solution talk.* New York: W.W. Norton.

Gillett, R. (1992). *Change your mind, change your world: A practical guide to turning limiting beliefs into positive realities.* New York: Simon and Schuster.

Kabat-Zinn, J. (1993). Meditation. In Bill Moyers (Ed.), *Healing and the mind* (pp. 115-143). New York: Doubleday.

Kerr, M. and Bowen, M. (1988). *Family evaluation: An approach based on Bowen theory.* New York: W.W. Norton.

Lee, J.A.B. (1994). *The empowerment approach to social work practice.* New York: Columbia University Press.

Lerner, M. (1993). Healing. In Bill Moyers (Ed.), *Healing and the mind* (pp. 323-341). New York: Doubleday.

Levine, S. (1987). *Healing into life and death.* New York: Anchor Doubleday.

Logan, S. (1994). *Reflections on creativity: Implications for an expanded perspective on social work practice.* Lawrence, KS: Hall Center for the Humanities.

Logan, S. (1996). *The black family: Strengths, self-help and positive change.* Boulder, CO: Westview.

Logan, S., Freeman, E., and McRoy, R. (Eds.) (1990). Social work practice with black families. New York: Longman, Inc.

Ogbu, J. and Fordham, S. (1986). Black students' success: Coping with the burden of acting white. *Urban Review, 18,* 176-206.

Remen, R.N. (1993). Wholeness. In Bill Moyers (Ed.), *Healing and the mind* (pp. 343-364). New York: Doubleday.

Reynolds, B.C. (1975). *Social work and social living.* New York: National Association of Social Workers.

Saleebey, D. (Ed.) (1992). *The strengths perspective in social work practice.* New York: Longman.

Schiele, J.H. (1996). Afrocentricity: An emerging paradigm in social work practice. *Social Work, 41*(3), 284-294.

Smalley, R.E. (1953). Mobilization of resources within the individual. *The Social Service Review, XXVIII*(3).

Smalley, R.E. (1958). Inner and outer resources that support the choice of life and growth. In *Proceedings, Conference on Social Crippling.* Baltimore, MD: State Department of Mental Health and the National Institute of Mental Health.

Smith, D. (1993). Healing and the community. In Bill Moyers (Ed.), *Healing and the mind* (pp. 47-64). New York: Doubleday.

Solomon, B. (1976). *Black empowerment social work in oppressed communities.* New York: Columbia University Press.

Swami Ananantanda (1996). *What's on my mind? Becoming inspired with new perception.* New York: SYDA Foundation.

Swami Chidvilasananda (1989). *Kindle my heart,* Volumes I and II. New York: SYDA Foundation.

Watzlawick, P., Weakland, J., and Fisch, R. (1974). *Change: The principles of problem formation and problem resolution.* New York: W.W. Norton.

White, M. and Epston, D. (1990). *Narrative means to therapeutic ends.* New York: Norton.

Chapter 10

Black Women and HIV/AIDS: Culturally Sensitive Family Health Care

Johnetta Miner

Historically, Americans of African ancestry have been a very proud group of people. As slaves they maintained a kind of connection and self-esteem through a sense of community and the extended family. Regardless of how poor the family might be, cleanliness and good personal hygiene were of the utmost importance. African-American families have had a very strong kinship bond and flexibility in roles within the family unit. Religion, education, and work are given great value. Self-esteem of this magnitude and quality has been a means of survival. Knowledge of this cultural diversity became part of the professional knowledge base in caring for HIV-positive African-American women. Professionals need to be cognizant of a number of psychosocial and cultural issues, as well as address them in their practices to meet the challenge of caring for these women and their families. This chapter describes a unique project that focused on ethnically appropriate health care interventions with HIV-positive African-American women and their families. The project successfully combined folk medicine and alternative therapies with traditional health care practices for African Americans in New York City, thus increasing the acceptance and effectiveness of traditional medical regimens.

HEALTH CARE NEEDS
OF AFRICAN-AMERICAN WOMEN WITH HIV/AIDS

African-American women, who make up more than half of the number of cases of women with AIDS, have not progressed as much as white women in the prevention and treatment of the disease. Although some progress has been made, African-American women still lack adequate knowledge regarding HIV/AIDS and equal access to treatment and research. It is of the utmost urgency that the helping professions advocate for this segment of the population. To advocate effectively, it is necessary for helping professionals to become more knowledgeable about the health care needs of African-American women.

Effective January 1, 1993, the Centers for Disease Control and Prevention (CDC) expanded the surveillance definition of AIDS to include those HIV-seropositive persons with CD4 T-lymphocyte counts below 200 cells or a CD4 percentage of total lymphocytes less than 14. In addition, three more diseases were added to the twenty-three AIDS indicator conditions of the previous definition. Included in the revised definition were pulmonary tuberculosis (TB), recurrent pneumonia, and invasive cervical cancer. This revised definition applies only to adults and adolescents (New York City Department of Health, 1993).

To be classified as recurrent pneumonia, two or more acute episodes of pneumonia must be diagnosed clinically within a twelve-month period. Radiological or laboratory tests are required to confirm the diagnoses. Pulmonary TB also requires clinical or culture confirmation. An increasing number of women have been diagnosed with AIDS according to the new definition; thus, the incidence of AIDS has increased overall in this population.

Among the individuals served by an urban hospital located in the borough of Queens in New York, 39.8 percent have incomes 200 percent below the federal poverty level, which impacts on their health care. Of this population, 16 percent are Medicaid eligible, as of January 1992, compared to 12.8 percent of the entire population within the borough of Queens. The hospital serves 27.4 percent of the borough's population, yet it serves 34.3 percent of the borough's Medicaid eligible population.

These factors, compounded by clients' positive HIV status, impact greatly on the health care needs and health-seeking behaviors of this population, and also on the health care rendered to this population. Statistics from CDC indicate that HIV is the leading cause of death in African-American women between the ages of twenty-five and forty. This mortality rate is correlated with increased cancer and heart disease rates among these women. Statistics indicate an increase in HIV-positive cases among black women age fifty and older. Suicides and homicides account for the fourth and fifth most common causes of death within this population, respectively. Along with the expanded definition of AIDS, an AIDS diagnosis implies hopelessness and death to many people, although they may be asymptomatic at the time. HIV and poverty among African-American women and their families are a lethal combination. Lack of culturally appropriate interventions for African-American families headed by women is a barrier to their seeking health care.

Within-Group Ethnic Diversity

Diversity exists among African-American families and communities. Single African-American families are not homogenous, contrary to stereotypes. Factors that create variations include religious backgrounds, socioeconomic status, geographic origins, age, and level of acculturation. Being black in the United States affects every aspect of family life and generates different coping strategies for individual families living with racism and discrimination on a daily basis. Clinicians need to be cautious about making generalizations about the health practices and lifestyles of black families, even among families from a given geographic region or from different regions, such as Alabama compared to the Carolinas, or northern states as opposed to southern states.

FAMILY AND GENDER STRESSORS AND SUPPORTS

Stressors

HIV infection in one family member affects all family members, especially female heads of households. The psychological and social impacts are compounded when both the mother and the child(ren) are seropositive. The mother will often secure health care for the child at her own expense, and many African-American women often admit that they have taken days off from work to follow up with their children's medical care. However, they neglect to do the same for themselves until they become ill. In addition, child care, accessible transportation, and adequate financial resources are other major issues of concern to HIV-infected African-American women. Furthermore, they fear stigmatization and rejection by family members. Women are often ambivalent about whether they should share information about their disease and their children's seropositive status. Family stress increases tenfold at a time when the immune system is already compromised by HIV. Many losses occur, including loss of health, employment, family members, friends, and economic independence. Roles within the family change, and the black female may no longer be the employed head of household but may assume the sick patient role while continuing to struggle to keep the family together.

Supports and Resources

Spiritual beliefs, relationships with extended family members, and faith are frequently renewed and strengthened as a means of coping. Strategies that have been utilized to cope with a racist society are also employed. Some clinicians may inaccurately assess strategies, such as denial and reticence, as depression or personality disorders.

Centuries of poverty, racism, oppression, and isolation, not being part of mainstream America, can lead to frustration, feelings of hopelessness, powerlessness, and, for some individuals, dependence on drugs and alcohol. However, as a group, African-American families are survivors, against all odds. They have retained a sense of pride. Traditionally, African-American families have had a very strong kinship bond and a flexibility in roles within the nuclear and extended family units. Religion, education, and work are given great value in black communities.

Black women still rely on kinship bonds that extend beyond blood lines as a coping strategy. "Aunts" and "uncles" may be individuals living next door who are not blood relatives. It should not be assumed that there is not a male role model in the home because the female client is single. Fathers and other male role models within the family need to be included in family treatment, disease prevention, and wellness promotion programs. Extended family members are an important aspect of family life. Some African-American females will seek health care more readily for their children than for themselves, and sooner than African-American males. Most African-American females are sicker when they seek health care than white women with HIV/AIDS because they cannot afford the cost or they put off seeking care because they do not feel ill. Historically, African-American women have been a strong force in the family, and some of them are willing to sacrifice themselves for the health and well-being of their families. They have shown tremendous empathy for the African-American males' feelings of frustration in a racist society, and they have often been wrongfully labeled as dominant matriarchs.

ACTP: A CULTURALLY SENSITIVE APPROACH TO WORKING WITH HIV-POSITIVE AFRICAN-AMERICAN WOMEN

The Population Served

The client population of the Alternative Co-Therapies Project (ACTP) is served within a large urban hospital in New York City. The hospital provides a range of services to Southeast Queens, which includes sixteen zip codes. Of the 1990 population served (535,597), approximately 20 percent were under the age of fifteen. Of this population, 45 percent were between the childbearing ages of fifteen and forty-four years. There was a higher percentage of females (53.6 percent) than males (46.4 percent) compared to the boroughwide (40 percent) and citywide (48 percent) female population. The majority of individuals receiving services are African American and Hispanic (67 percent). Many of them are suspicious of Western white medicine; therefore, a user-friendly approach was needed to address the specific concerns of African-American females.

The Project's Goals

The ACTP goals were to develop approaches that were culturally sensitive to the health care needs of HIV-positive African-American women and their families and that would help meet their specific ethnic needs. These approaches need to address clients' socioeconomic status, as their ability to meet their basic needs influences their health status. As Hines and Boyd-Franklin (1982) have noted, it is important that clinicians on the frontlines of HIV/AIDS health care services utilize all the strengths and resources that can be mobilized to assist black women and their families. The objectives of the project included the following:

1. To gain patients' trust. Clinicians must first gain the trust of the individual and assess that person's coping strategies without making generalizations. Gaining trust is easier for culturally sensitive clinicians because they use an ethnosensitive knowledge base.
2. To provide counseling and alternative treatments that are unique to the ethnic requirements of the target population.
3. To incorporate a holistic approach within the counseling process and traditional treatment regimen that includes folk medicine and alternative/cotherapies such as herbs and massage.
4. To make comprehensive social, physical, and mental health assessments that also take family and ethnic issues into consideration.
5. To utilize all the strengths and resources that can be mobilized to assist African-American women and their families in meeting their health care needs.
6. To include fathers and male figures of the family in family treatment, disease prevention, and wellness promotion systems, as the patient allows.
7. To eliminate generalizations about the lifestyles of African-American families because there is a great diversity within this ethnic group, depending on socioeconomic status, geographic origin, level of acculturation, age, and religious background.

The Importance of Taking a Sexual History

Further, the project's experience underscores the need for a more comprehensive assessment. Given that women as a group have been less likely to be identified with HIV than men, it is imperative that health care professionals expand their approach in assessing and providing services to this population. The need is evident in the increasing rate of heterosexual transmission of HIV/AIDS as compared to other modes of transmission. During assessments, sexual histories of women should be taken at all points of entry to the health care system, including inner-city emergency rooms, community health centers, and family planning and obstetrical settings. These assessments should be conducted in a culturally sensitive manner as a part of the first contact with African-American women, regardless of the setting. It is important to recognize that patients, as well as providers, are reluctant to discuss sexual practices and histories due to their discomfort about such subject matter. Obtaining a sexual history needs to be a routine part of recording a medical history. The interviewer should set the stage by not making assumptions or implying judgments about any client's history. For example, the interviewer should ask, "Do you have sex with men, women, or both?" as opposed to "Are you gay, lesbian, or bisexual?" Interviewers should try to determine the patient's level of understanding about sexual matters. The question regarding sexual practices may need to be clarified as to what is meant by the word *sex.* Sex to one female may mean vaginal intercourse, while to another it may mean oral sex. Sexual history taking requires time and cannot be circumvented by making assumptions.

Questions to include in the sexual history taking are as follows:

1. Are you sexually active?
2. Do you have sex with men, women, or both?
3. How many sexual partners have you had in the past six months?
4. How many men? How many women?
5. What kind of sex do you have? Oral? Anal? Vaginal?
6. Do you ever have sex without a condom?
7. Have you or any of your sexual partners ever injected drugs or medications?
8. Have you ever had a sexually transmitted disease? What was it? When? Was it treated? With what medication? For how long?
9. Do you have a vaginal discharge? Have you been having vaginal discharges or burning upon urination?
10. Are you pregnant?
11. Do you practice birth control? What method?

12. What are the family's sexual practices that can be viewed as secrets (e.g., incest, rape, physical abuse, etc.)?

These questions are suggested as guidelines for incorporating sensitivity into the process of assessing and intervening with African-American women and their families. In addition, it is necessary to institute a plan of action during intake to inform patients of their test results in case they neglect to return for follow-up care.

This project (ACTP) has implemented a number of interrelated steps in health education, disease prevention, and wellness promotion. Often HIV-positive women are distrustful of treatment, not only because of various incidents in which black Americans were unwillingly and unknowingly exploited and harmed in government experiments and projects, but also because of their distrust of traditional Western ethnocentric medicine. Some African-American patients prefer folk medicine and alternative/cotherapies such as vitamins, micronutrients, herbs, acupuncture, and massage (see Table 10.1). Project staff respect these preferences and explore whether clients want them included with the traditional treatment regimen. A vast amount of knowledge can be gained from these patients, as many of them rely on their faith and the powerful connection between their body, mind, and spirit.

The ACTP's Services

This project's experience demonstrates that culturally appropriate comprehensive family health care should include the following services:

1. Child care
2. Transportation or money for transportation
3. Money or monetary tokens as incentives for clinic attendance and keeping appointments
4. Appointments for different family members on the same day during the same time period
5. Comprehensive health care services such as HIV/AIDS, OB/GYN, pediatrics, primary medical care, dental, and dermatology to be provided in the same building
6. Alternative/cotherapies
7. Culturally competent clinicians

TABLE 10.1. Alternative/Cotherapies

Micronutrients	Antioxidants	Therapies	Teas
Calcium Magnesium Potassium Iron	CoQ10 Vitamins A, C, E Zinc Selenium Beta-carotene	Physical therapy Exercise Relaxation methods Massage Acupuncture Guided imagery Visualization Touch therapy	Commercial herb teas Chamomile Hibiscus Peppermint Ginger Tilo
Symptom-Specific Therapies				
Fatigue Ginseng Bee pollen Astralgus *Thrush/Vaginal Yeast* Lactobacillus Acidophilus Garlic Echinacea Astralgus	*Dry Skin* Vitamin E oil Peanut oil Systemic vitamin E Petroleum jelly Keri lotion	*Stress* B-complex C-complex Bee pollen	*Antiviral/Anti-inflammatory* Ascorbic acid Garlic Goldenseal Burdock Echinacea Zinc	*Nasal Congestion Postnasal Drip* Warm saline water Garlic Carrot juice Beta-carotene Saline nasal wash Bee pollen Vitamin C Zinc Reduce intake of mucus-forming foods Thyme

A Case Example

This case example illustrates the project's culturally appropriate, comprehensive cotherapies and family services. The case involves a thirty-six-year-old African-American female who was admitted to the antepartum unit of the hospital with a right axillary cyst that had opened two weeks prior to admission and again on the day of admission. Originally, she had been referred to the emergency room by a pediatric social worker who noticed the patient had a draining breast mass. She was considered a high-risk pregnancy at thirty-two weeks' gestation and had been diagnosed HIV positive in 1991. One initial visit had been made to the medical infectious disease clinic six months after diagnosis. She reported no prenatal care and thought she was at twenty-five weeks' gestation. Her past medical history revealed an STD, anemia, left ovarian cyst, S/P (superficial perianal) repair of a perianal abscess, and substance use (smoked crack and marijuana). Admission findings included a positive toxicology for marijuana, VDRL reactive 1:1, breast mass, and a CD4 count of 236.

The patient had an eleventh-grade education and was receiving welfare assistance. There was a family history of cancer. All of her children were in foster care or adopted. Her last child, a two-year-old HIV-positive male, was admitted to the pediatric unit at the same time as the patient's admission. A sixteen-year-old son who had "run away" from adoptive parents was living with the patient. This son was reported to have a behavior problem. The father of this current pregnancy was incarcerated, charged by the patient, for family violence. The patient had periodic contact with a sibling living in the South and no contact with other siblings. Both parents were deceased.

Referral was made by the medical service to the HIV/AIDS service for follow-up and possible treatment. A nursing referral was also made to the same service for psychiatric nursing assessment, HIV/AIDS education, HIV/AIDS nursing assessment, and cotherapies.

Multidisciplinary team interventions. The patient was seen by the attending physician for HIV/AIDS care and the recommendation was not to treat the patient with antiretroviral therapy in light of her pregnant status and the more prominent diagnosis of breast cancer. The patient was also seen by this clinician for assessment.

The patient was alert and oriented to person, place, and time. Her cognitive process was slow and HIV information needed to be repeated. No changes were noted in her mental state, and there were no indications of depression. Her mood was sad, which was attributed to her overwhelming concern for her son, whom she had been visiting on the pediatric unit. Her concern was viewed as a positive factor because it directed her attention away from herself.

It was decided that she would benefit from imagery and nutritional support since she was primarily an oncology patient. The nurse practitioner recommended nutritional supplements, such as vitamin C, B-complex, prenatal vitamins, and Sustacal; ongoing psychiatric and emotional support; initiation of visiting nurse services for home care follow-up; pain management, since the patient complained of severe pain; and social work intervention for herself, her children, and the unborn baby. The patient wanted to retain custody of her son and unborn child.

Seven days after admission, her membranes ruptured and she was transferred to obstetrics. Three days later she delivered a four-pound, five-ounce daughter, and was transferred to a unit for post-partum care, where she signed out against medical advice.

She later returned to the oncology clinic for follow-up care, at which time consultation was made with the clinic nurse regarding her need for care since she had signed out before any therapeutic interventions could be instituted. The patient was readmitted for chemotherapy and HIV nursing intervention, such as continued education, emotional support, and visualization techniques.

She received two cycles of treatment with Cytoxan and 5FU (5-fluorouracil), emotional support, continued education, and visualization techniques. Her appetite was poor to fair, she had periods of nausea and vomiting, and her CD4 count had stabilized at approximately 363. The cancerous tumor of the breast had enlarged. Continuous communication was made with social service regarding her need for home care services, such as a registered nurse, aide, transportation, and feedback in reference to the outcome of the placement of her young son. The patient was followed throughout her hospitalization on various units, and emotional support and coordination for services was provided throughout. There was continuous contact with the social service department. Clear communication across disciplines and with nursing staff was a crucial part of the treatment plan.

On a subsequent visit to the HIV/AIDS clinic, a change in the patient's behavior was noted. The patient was very talkative, volunteering information, and was constantly moving about in her chair. A urine toxicology was requested, and the results returned were positive for cocaine and other illicit agents.

Thereafter, the case went before the tumor board, and the decision was to treat the tumor with Taxol and G-CSF (granulocyte colony stimulating factor), which resulted in a decrease in tumor size. No antiretroviral therapy was recommended. However, the patient was lost to treatment and attempts to contact her by telephone were unsuccessful. A telephone call was made to the visiting nurse, who had conversed with her a few seconds prior to my calling. The patient was informed about the success of the Taxol treatment and the need to return to the oncology and immunology clinics for follow-up care and counseling. Not only did the patient return to the clinics but she also returned for hospitalization for chemotherapy.

Nursing interventions. The clinical nurse specialist on the antepartum unit followed through on the various recommendations and initiated the following referrals: dietary for adequate nutrition/nutritional counseling and supplementation; visiting nurse and home care service following discharge; and pediatric for visitation of son. Referral was also made by this nurse for pastoral counseling and spiritual support, social service intervention, immunology team for additional ongoing support, and doctor's orders for cotherapies and initial analgesic for pain management.

Nursing interventions were aimed at strengthening the flexible lines of defense and the lines of resistance in addition to maintaining system stability. The intervention strategies were tertiary in nature and included the following:

1. HIV/AIDS education
2. Behavior modification: history of substance use
3. Development of realistic view of seriousness of illnesses
4. Use of available resources
5. Wound care for alteration in skin integrity and universal precautions
6. Assessment for adequate pain management
7. Treatment for anxiety related to diagnoses, lack of prior follow-up care, and separation from son
8. Assistance in retaining and maintaining coping strategies (she focused on her son, turned inward, and presented a very simple and honest demeanor)
9. Application of a culturally sensitive, holistic approach to nursing interventions. (Miner, 1995)

CONCLUSION

African-American women, such as the one in the previous case example, were very receptive to culturally sensitive health care combined with cotherapies. As a result of such culturally sensitive health care, they are often more receptive to traditional medical practices as well. The return rates to the clinic increased among patients, and the medical staff requested information about alternative therapies and African-American culture, and made direct referrals to the nurse clinician for counseling. The diversity among ethnic/racial groups, such as regional differences, level of acculturation, and health behaviors, affects an individual's health care and health outcomes. Cultural values, which are related to ethnicity, community, and family, play an important role in meeting the health care needs of HIV-positive African-American women and families. Although some of the suggestions for comprehensive family health services and incorporating sensitivity into the interviewing and assessment process are applicable to all women, they are especially recommended for African-American women. Interviews revealed that many of these women were not receiving such services in other programs simply because they were African American.

The approach utilized during interviewing and counseling of these patients may be compared to NTU (pronounced "in-to") psychotherapy, a spiritually based Afrocentric approach. The principles of NTU therapy include cultural awareness, authenticity, interconnectedness, harmony, and balance (Phillips, 1990). According to Phillips (1990), NTU is the basic element that unifies the universe, and, as such, it is the essence of life. The NTU concept can certainly be applied to education and practice through the incorporation of cultural sensitivity for meeting the health care needs of HIV-positive African-American women.

ACTP has direct implications for HIV/AIDS prevention programs, clinical practice, and nursing, medical, and social work education, in addition to designing and conducting social and medical research with African-American patients in the HIV/AIDS arena.

REFERENCES

Hines, P.M. and Boyd-Franklin, N. (1982). Black families. In M. McGoldrick, J.K. Pearce, and J. Giordano (Eds.), *Ethnicity and family therapy* (pp. 108-122). New York: The Guilford Press.

Miner, J. (1995). Incorporating the Betty Neuman Systems Model into HIV clinical practice. *AIDS Patient Care*, February, 36-39.

New York City Department of Health (1993). The revised AIDS case definition. *CHI City Health Information, 12*(1) (February 1), 1.

Phillips, F.B. (1990). NTU psychology: An Afrocentric approach. *The Journal of Black Psychology, 17*(1), 55-74.

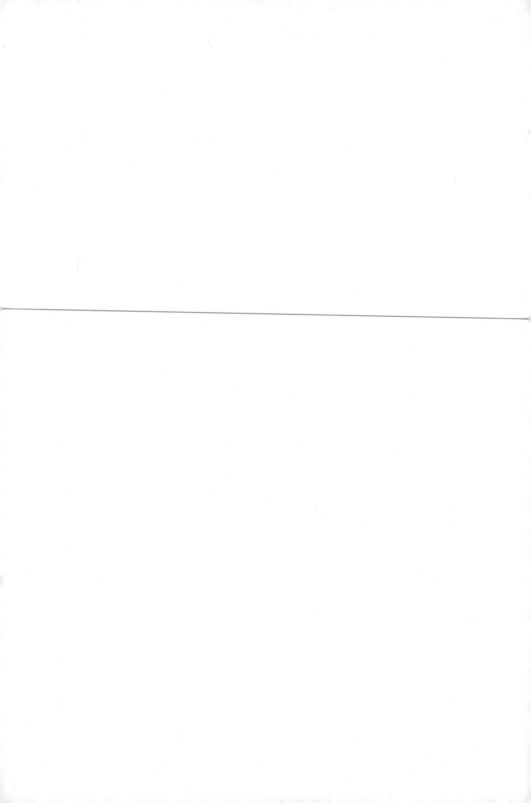

Chapter 11

The Black Church Response
to the Mental Health Needs
of the Elderly

Freda Brashears

A discussion of community-based mental health service delivery to African Americans would not be complete without acknowledging the unique and prominent role of the church in African-American culture. It is generally agreed that the church has had an impact upon virtually every aspect of African-American life and is central to the experience of being black in America (Taylor, Thornton, and Chatters, 1987). In addition to spiritual sustenance provided through a set of core beliefs, the church has a long history of providing social services to members of the African-American community. It has been a particularly reliable vehicle for providing services to elderly African Americans (Coke and Twaite, 1995).

Records dating to 1914 indicate that it is common for the church to "supply all needs of the community at the church" (Ross, 1978, p. 243), and for members to reach out into the community to "care for . . . all that are needy" (Ross, 1978, p. 411). The black church has established schools, orphanages, senior citizen homes, and social and recreational centers for young people and adults. It has also been called upon to provide health and mental health services to the African-American community.

Secular agencies recognize that the church is a force to join with as well as a place to provide direct service to African Americans (Hatch and Derthick, 1992). Successful service delivery collaboration between African-American churches and secular agencies is found in many communities (Thomas et al., 1994). Health promotion activities regarding a variety of issues have shown positive results in both inner-city urban and rural community churches when presented with culturally specific intervention strategies (Stillman et al., 1993; Sutherland, Hale, and Harris, 1995; Turner et al., 1995). Mental health services offered through church-based programs in the African-American community are often accepted by secular agency professionals as being complementary rather than competitive (Ambrose, 1976; Lyles, 1992).

The church plays a particularly significant role in the lives of elderly African-American people. Of African-American adults over fifty-five years of age, 80 percent identify themselves as church members (Taylor, 1993). For elderly African Americans, there is significant association between their involvement in church and their physical as well as mental health. They report that they perceive God in a very personal way and consider God to be as much a part of their informal support system as are family, friends, or neighbors (Taylor and Chatters, 1986; Wood and Wan, 1993).

African Americans over sixty years of age and across all levels of income, education, and occupation report that because of their spiritual beliefs and church activities, they are able to cope and have life satisfaction in spite of advanced age, social problems related to their race, or poverty (Benton, 1988; Ellison, 1997; Johnson, 1995; Krause, 1992; Nye, 1992; Smith, 1993). Older African Americans frequently state that a major coping strategy for them is prayer (Taylor, 1993; Wilson-Ford, 1992) and that participation in church communities reduces stress, increases positive self-esteem, and leads to living healthier lifestyles (Brown and Gary, 1994; Coke and Twaite, 1995; Ellison, 1993, 1997; Taylor, 1993; Walls, 1992). The African-American church is clearly a significant source of emotional and social support for older African Americans.

This chapter explores the historical development of the African-American church and the role it plays in African-American culture and mental health. A brief outline of the theology that shapes the core religious and spiritual beliefs is given, and a case example is presented that illustrates the application of those beliefs to the mental health needs of the African-American elderly. It concludes with implications for social work practice.

HISTORY OF THE AFRICAN-AMERICAN CHURCH

Organized African-American churches date from at least 1773, with congregations in both northern and southern states. In the early days of the colonies, attempts were made to Christianize the Africans brought to America as slaves. Evangelical preachers sought their conversion and encouraged Africans to learn English ways including the language and the religion. Slaveowners taught a religion that considered slavery to be the will of God and allowed their slaves to attend their own churches under the watchful eye of the overseer. In northern states, it was common for African Americans and American whites to attend church together, as long as they sat separately and African Americans were not allowed to lead or actively partake in the services along with the Caucasian members (Coke and Twait, 1995).

In 1794, a group of free African Americans in Philadelphia broke away from the American white Methodist Episcopal Church and formed the African Methodist Episcopal Church. Baptist churches formed about the same time, and by 1840, enough of them existed to form a national organization at the Abyssinian Baptist Church in Harlem. Baptist churches tended to be composed of slaves or freedmen, while African Methodist Episcopal churches tended to be composed more of freemen (Jones and Matthews, 1976).

Slaves in the South began to believe in the teachings of their Caucasian Christian preachers and identified themselves with the Old Testament Children of Israel in Egyptian bondage waiting to be set free. Some began to speak up for their freedom, and some became preachers for their own slave communities. Some led unsuccessful revolts against the slave society. After such rebellions, even more severe restrictions were placed on slave communities. Those restrictions included all gatherings, especially religious services. As a result, slave churches became "invisible communities of faith" (Costen, 1993), and worship took whatever form was possible. One such form was the music that has become known as the traditional Negro spiritual (Sanger, 1995; Thurman, 1975). In spite of everything, African Americans and their churches survived into modern times.

THE ROLE OF THE CHURCH
IN AFRICAN-AMERICAN CULTURE

African Americans are said to be the most religious group in the world. A national poll by Gallup and Castelli (1991) found that 81 percent of African Americans were church members, 78 percent believed religion was important in their personal lives, and 93 percent felt that religion would become even more important to them over the next five years. Coke and Twaite (1995) found in the National Study of African Americans that 78 percent prayed daily and 71 percent attended church at least once per month. Smith (1993) reported that African Americans of all occupations, incomes, and educational levels actively participate in organizational activities in the church.

The Gallup poll also found that even though a large majority reported church membership, evidence suggested that religious knowledge was limited to less than 65 percent. Gallup concluded that the discrepancy between the percentages of church membership and religious knowledge could be attributed to the relatively low percentage of college graduates among African Americans. By looking for association between church membership and religious knowledge, Gallup implies that a primary reason for church membership or attendance is to gain such knowledge. However, it is possible to draw alternative conclusions from these data.

One conclusion could be that African Americans belong to and attend church for reasons other than, or in addition to, religious education. The church has performed many functions throughout history besides religious ones. When access to dominant-culture institutions and services were denied them, African Americans turned to one another. The church often served as a place to meet, where members of the community could pass the news, take care of business, and find strength of purpose.

The church has often provided direct social welfare services as well as leadership for social activism. It was part of the Underground Railroad during slavery, for example, and provided secular education and other social services to African Americans when they were unavailable from any other source (Allen-Meares, 1989; McAdoo and Crawford, 1991). The church was a stabilizing force in the days after emancipation when it provided leadership to newly freed slaves in a manner that Du Bois (in Pollard, 1978) character-ized as being similar to the social structure of ancient tribal cultures in which religious leaders offered guidance and reassurance to the people. The church continued to provide refuge as well as a moral compass for African Americans during the turbulent civil rights struggles of the twentieth century.

The significance of the church may be attributed to its position as one of the few institutions in the African-American community that is primarily built, financed, and controlled by African Americans (Taylor, Thornton, and Chatters, 1987). Leadership positions denied in the larger community are available in the church. The church may also be one of the few institutions that is owned by African Americans, in the psychological sense of ownership, in that it repre-sents black culture itself. The African-American church serves as a transmitter of cultural history that is unique among religious organi-zations. Through its rituals and traditions, cultural awareness and history of the African-American experience are taught. Individual, family, and cultural identities are learned in the church.

Although reference to the African-American church as if it were a single organization to which all African Americans belong is inaccu-rate, the church as a cultural experience is an index of African-Amer-ican community identification. The national surveys mentioned earli-er indicate that the experience of church is common to many, and some suggest that religion may be the closest thing there is to a corporate African-American identity (Lincoln, 1995). Religious ori-entation is considered to be one of the greatest strengths of African-American families (Coke and Twait, 1995; Dancy and Wynn-Dancy, 1994).

The African-American church and its religious tradition are unique to African Americans. It is the way it is, in part, because African-American people over the centuries have experienced God and their worship of God in the light of their continual suffering (Dash, Jackson, and Rasor, 1997). Formed in the midst of slavery, and continually shaped by the oppression of Jim Crow segregation, discrimination, and institutional racism, the church provides for African Americans the means for coping and surviving in a hostile world (Morris and Robinson, 1996; Washington, 1994). James

Baldwin is said to have observed that African Americans would lose all their minds if it were not for religion and the African-American church (Stewart, 1997). Richard Wright (1941, p. 131) describes the African-American church as the place "where we dip our tired bodies in the cool springs of hope, where we retain our wholeness and humanity despite the blows of death."

Theology of the African-American Church

The theology of the African-American church is rooted in African religious tradition (Coke and Twaite, 1995; Dash, Jackson, and Rasor, 1997; Sobel, 1988; Stewart, 1997). In that tradition, all parts of this and other-world existence are associated with acts of a Supreme Deity who is believed to have created and maintains a well-ordered, balanced, and harmonious universe. In that balanced and harmonious universe, life is viewed by the believer as being holistic, with all events being related to, or controlled by, acts of God. In this belief system, all persons, experiences, and events are considered to be sacred, with no separation or compartmentalizing between sacred and secular areas of life (Costen, 1993).

The African tradition was brought to North America with slavery, where it met Judeo-Christian religion and the particular practice of European-American Christianity, as presented by Evangelical preachers during the slave era. The Christian tradition taught that God and Jesus are one and the same in the Holy Trinity. It taught that God could be known at a personal level through the belief and acceptance of Jesus Christ as the Son of God who died and rose again to save souls from eternal damnation as well as from the despairs of this world.

The two religious traditions fit together for Africans in America. The Christian belief that Jesus can be a personal savior blended with the African belief that God can be known personally and not just known about from doctrines or creeds (Costen, 1993). The Christian message that Jesus was a deliverer of disinherited and oppressed people was particularly meaningful to African slaves in America (Thurman, 1976). The pressure of slavery melded the two traditions together.

An early African-American folk religion known as the Jesus-faith emerged from the blended traditions. Characterized as an Africanization of Christianity (Walker, 1976), the Jesus-faith was an everyday religion with a holistic theology that taught that God continually intervenes to provide health, strength, and joy. It was a religion in which spirituality was lived in daily life, with no aspect of life being outside its realm (Costen, 1993). Slave life deepened the need for such an everyday religion and belief that God would preserve even through the most horrible of times.

The religion of African Americans, blended from African and American Christian traditions, tempered and shaped by the slave experience, grew into a belief system, or faith. That belief system preserves the African understanding of the spirituality of reality and adds the Christian understanding of Jesus and individual salvation (Sobel, 1988). It does not distinguish between science, or reason, and faith. All things, including the supernatural, were included in it (Mitchell, 1972). That belief system or faith has distinct meanings, beliefs, and practices that continue into modern times and is unique to African Americans. It provides the spiritual sustenance needed still for African Americans to survive, intact, against all odds, and to have a meaningful existence in spite of harsh social and political circumstances and the concerted efforts by others to deny it.

The basic distinction of the African-American Christian tradition is an unyielding faith in the absolute sovereignty of a Supreme Infinite Creator known as God (King, 1972). The core beliefs of that tradition are described by Cooper-Lewter and Mitchell (1986):

1. God is in charge of the universe and all that is within it.
2. God is sovereign and omnipotent with unlimited control and power.
3. God knows everything, is just, impartial, and fair.
4. God is gracious, always forgiving, with unconditional, unmerited acceptance.
5. Each person is unique and worthy of respect, and all people are intrinsically equal.
6. People can and should endure in their identity and faith.
7. All black people are related as family.

This set of core beliefs appears to be generalized throughout African-American culture. It translates into what is referred to as the "Black Church." The Black Church is more than an organizational entity defined by doctrine and worship practices. It and its worship traditions have become a way of living for African Americans. It represents an applied theology by which life experiences are faced, with faith in a God who is known at the personal level and who is in control of all aspects of living, for both the individual and the larger community.

The spiritual support provided by this set of core beliefs contributes to the general mental well-being of all members of the African-American church as they are applied to everyday life situations. The beliefs provide a way for people to make sense of traumatic life events. They teach that God cares about individuals and what happens to them even before an event occurs, thus providing a buffer against stress and contributing to wellness. The spiritual beliefs teach that individuals can receive support directly from their own relationship to God, independent of support from others such as church members, the pastor, family, or friends (Westgate, 1996). Acting upon their beliefs, African Americans consider God to be a part of their total support system and expect to receive instrumental support and respite from God (Wood and Wan, 1993). The essence of African-American spirituality has its roots in African traditions and in faith, which is reflected in the set of core beliefs discussed by Cooper-Lewter and Mitchell (1986).

A Case Example: Second Baptist Church,
Kansas City, Missouri

Second Baptist Church in Kansas City, Missouri, provides a microcosmic example of the African-American Church in America. Born of slaves, under the trees of a riverbank, nurtured through the generations by its faithful members, it has lived the entire life of African Americans since freedom. It teaches the core beliefs and proactively applies them to daily living. It epitomizes the African-American experience in America.

Second Baptist is the oldest African-American church in Kansas City, Missouri. It was founded in October 1863, just ten months after the signing of the Emancipation Proclamation, by a group of people that surely included recently freed slaves. This group started a mission at a spot on the banks of the Missouri River called Straggler's Camp. Having no building, the group worshipped under the trees, just as slaves in southern states had always done in their invisible communities of faith (Hunter, 1940). From that beginning, Second Baptist has had an unbroken history for 135 years. Its members like to say their church may be the Second Baptist Church in town, but it is second to none in its importance to them and the community.

In the 135 years since Straggler's Camp, Second Baptist has had three locations and seven pastors. The first building, valued at $100,000, was completed in 1898, a remarkable feat considering the journey of Reconstruction in the slave state of Missouri and the newly enacted Jim Crow laws of the early 1890s. The new building was just ten blocks from the camp on the Missouri River bank. It was a magnificently large building that could seat hundreds of people at a time and had a pipe organ that was described as the best in the city. The National Baptist Convention held its annual meeting at Second Baptist Church in the first year it was open (Payne, 1983).

. The splendor of the first church home was not to last, however. The building was destroyed by fire on a Saturday night in the spring of 1926. The membership attempted to rebuild in 1928 but were caught in the throes of the Depression. Until 1941, the congregation, not giving up its faith or its hope, and knowing from the history of its people that worship can occur anywhere under any circumstances, adverse or not, met in what was to have been the basement of the new church. At that time, not able to pay the mortgage on even that rudiment of a building, Second Baptist was assisted by a Caucasian congregation to purchase another building, one more similar to their first one.

The Caucasian congregation had a majestic "four-story modern, fully-equipped building complete with a library, gymnasium, pipe organ, grand pianos, oaken benches and broadloom carpeting" (Payne, 1983, p. 28). It was about ten blocks from Second Baptist. It appears that the Caucasian congregation planned to move out of the increasingly black neighborhood and made Second Baptist a very good deal on their building.

Being African American, people who had always been adept at making good use of things that Caucasian people did not want anymore, Second Baptist bought the building and continued to provide spiritual and social support to its members and the surrounding

community for the next twenty-two years. At that time, they pur-
chased a newer building, thirty-nine blocks from the river. The
newer building was available for purchase because its previous
congregation of Caucasian people was moving out of the now increasingly black neighborhood (Payne, 1983). Again, it was the
second Baptist church created, but being second to none, it continues to the present day as the primary source of sustenance to all who
enter, exemplifying the core belief that identity and faith should be
preserved.

Applying the core belief that all African Americans are related as
family, Second Baptist views itself as a large family system whose
needs are met within itself, and where all aspects of living are
recognized and supported. Following the tradition of African-
American churches throughout history (Pollard, 1978; Ross, 1978),
it has long cared for its members. In 1911, the Relief Workers Club
was organized "to assist in the care of unfortunate members of the
church" (Payne, 1983, p. 15). In 1925, the church organized the
Ever Ready Girls Club to promote growth in Christian character
and service through physical, social, and spiritual training. There is
a Birthday, Travel, Health, and Happiness Club through which
health fitness, social activities, and group travel tours are arranged.
The church sponsors recreation teams for youths, Boy Scout troops,
after-school tutorial programs, and social activities for all ages.
Concrete social services are delivered to members of the church and
the community through the church's social services department. An
additional social service ministry was developed several years ago
to meet the particular needs of elderly members who were facing
health crisis and terminal illness (Brashears and Roberts, 1996).

*Second Baptist's Response to the Mental Health Needs
of Its Elderly Members*

The congregation of Second Baptist Church has become increasingly more aged over the past two decades, a common experience
among many churches (Doka, 1986). Over the past ten years, more
than 100 longtime members and central leaders of the church have
died. The number of deaths seems to increase every year. Because
of this phenomenon, greater demand was placed on the pastor to
provide services.

In response to the demand, Second Baptist added a master's level social worker to the staff to assist in caring for the mental health and general well-being of elderly members who were experiencing distress, health crises, and death. The social worker developed a generalist practice of case management, general support services to homebound or institutionalized elderly members and their families, and individual and family counseling that incorporated the spiritual belief system of the church.

The social worker was a member of the church who shared the faith beliefs of others in the congregation and supported the church's traditional role of providing leadership and social services to the black community. Because African religious tradition still directs the lives of African-American people and their churches, a variation of the usual worker-client relationship developed that blended the professional self with the personal self and the secular education with religious and spiritual beliefs. While adhering to the strictest professional ethics of client self-determination and confidentiality, but with no artificial identities or assigned roles of worker or client, the social worker was able to draw from both professional training and the set of shared beliefs to provide ministry as well as service to members of the church and their families.

Case management services focused on preventing institutional placement by participating in discharge planning from the hospital and arranging for in-home services from community resources as well as the various ministries of the church. Support to homebound and institutionalized members was given through extensive field visits. In addition, the social worker arranged for individual church members or church groups to "adopt" shut-in members for frequent and regular friend-to-friend visiting and holiday remembrance. These services, while using sound social work principles and techniques, were specifically structured to draw from the belief that all African Americans are related as family and rely on each other through systems of mutual aid and informal support.

Another component of the social work practice was individual and family counseling with persons who were experiencing health crises and terminal illness. The counseling work focused on grief and loss issues as well as on helping the person and family prepare for living with illness, preparing for imminent death, and living through the experience of dying. A central part of the counseling service drew upon the core beliefs of the omnipotence of God, the all-knowing nature of God, a God who is just and fair, and a God who is known on a personal basis. Member clients did not ignore the power and remedies of medical science, but their ultimate faith and source of strength was their unyielding belief in the sovereignty of a God who is in charge of all things, great and small.

CONCLUSION

The social service program and ministry was instituted at Second Baptist Church in direct response to the mental health needs of elderly members who were experiencing what can be described as the ultimate life crisis. Its conception and implementation emanated from the traditional history of the church and its role in African-American culture and drew from and upon the core beliefs and faith of African-American Christianity. Its implications for social work practice are many.

The social work profession's understanding of human behavior can be enhanced, broadened, and deepened by using an African-American perspective that includes the spiritual beliefs found in black culture in America. The belief system speaks to human behavior phenomena, such as adaptation to, and resiliency from, life's struggles, acceptance of circumstances and forgiveness toward others who may have done wrong, and the reassurance that there is an ultimate justice.

The spiritual beliefs of African-American culture often serve as the ultimate coping mechanism for elderly persons when they are living through health crises. For example, because the African-American spiritual tradition believes that all life events are connected in a harmonious and balanced world, single events such as ill health may be considered part of a larger life narrative, one that has been turned over to the Lord, the source of all healing (Potts, 1996).

African-American spiritual belief does not separate the mind or spirit from the body, as modern medical practice seems to do. Therefore, social work practice approaches that use a medical model dualism are likely to be less effective with African-American clients. Those clients may consider the religious or spiritual side of their care more important than the medical approach. Social workers who address spiritual and cultural dimensions of the issues at hand are likely to develop more appropriate and effective therapeutic relationships and psychosocial interventions with their elderly African-American clients.

Social work practice can also be enhanced when the belief that all African Americans are related as family is incorporated into psychosocial intervention planning. This belief is manifest in the black community through the use of informal supports and mutual aid in responding to individual and family needs. Social workers developing care plans for institutionalized clients or preparing discharge plans for hospitalized clients should recognize and accept this service resource as the powerful one that it is. It should be considered as a first-order source of service rather than as a fallback when other resources fail.

Social workers who recognize that the church plays a multifaceted role in the African-American community phenomenon and bring it into their helping relationships will have taken a step toward providing culturally sensitive and appropriate service. The church represents more than the very visible role of political and social activist leader and more than a provider of concrete services to the general community. It represents the essence, or soul, of African-American culture. For its members, the church and its set of beliefs are often considered to be more important and powerful sources of healing than any other. A wise social worker who intends to be culturally competent will make active use of the black church in the provision of mental health services to elderly African Americans.

REFERENCES

Allen-Meares, P. (1989). Adolescent sexuality and premature parenthood: Role of the black church in prevention. *Journal of Social Work and Human Sexuality, 8*(19), 133, 142.

Ambrose, J.J (1976). The black church as a mental health resource. In D.J. Jones and W.H. Matthews (Eds.), *The black church: A community resource for urban affairs and research* (pp. 105-113). Washington, DC: Howard University.

Benton, B. (1988). Religion and cultural values: Neglected dimensions of life satisfaction measurements of black elderly poor. *Social Work and Christianity, 15*(2), 69-86.

Brashears, F. and Roberts, M. (1996). The black church as a resource for change. In S. Logan (Ed.), *The black family: Strengths, self-help and positive change* (pp. 181-192). Boulder, CO: Westview Press.

Brown, D.R. and Gary, L.E. (1994). Religious involvement and health status among African-American males. *Journal of the National Medical Association, 86*(11), 825-831.

Coke, M.M. and Twaite, J.A. (1995). *The black elderly: Satisfaction and quality of later life.* Binghamton, NY: The Haworth Social Work Practice Press.

Cooper-Lewter, N.C. and Mitchell, H.H. (1986). *Soul theology: The heart of American black culture.* San Francisco: Harper & Row.

Costen, M.W. (1993). *African American Christian worship.* Nashville, TN: Abingdon Press.

Dancy, J. and Wynn-Dancy, M.L. (1994). Faith of our fathers (mothers) living still: Spirituality as a force for the transmission of family values within the black community. *Activities, Adaptation, and Aging, 19*(2), 86-105.

Dash, M.I.N., Jackson, J., and Rasor, S.C. (1997). *Hidden wholeness: An African-American spirituality for individuals and communities.* Cleveland, OH: United Church Press.

Doka, K.J. (1986). The church and the elderly: The impact of changing age strata on congregations. *International Journal of Aging and Human Development, 22*(4), 291-300.

Ellison, C.G. (1993). Religious involvement and self-perception among black Americans. *Social Forces, 71*(4), 1027-1055.

Ellison, C.G. (1997). Religious involvement and the subjective quality of life among African Americans. In R.J. Taylor, J.S. Jackson, and L.M. Chatters (Eds.), *Family life in black America* (pp. 117-131). Thousand Oaks, CA: Sage Publications, Inc.

Gallup, G., Jr., and Castelli, J. (1991). Religious activity of blacks is up. *The Kansas City Star,* June 8, E-11.

Hatch, J. and Derthick, S. (1992). Empowering black churches for health promotion. *Health Values: The Journal of Health Behavior, Education, and Promotion, 16*(5), 3-9.

Hunter, J.E. (1940). *A nickel and a prayer.* Cleveland, OH: Elli Kani Publishing Company.

Johnson, C.L. (1995). Determinants of adaptation of oldest old black Americans. *Journal of Aging Studies, 9*(3), 231-244.

Jones, D.J. and Matthews, W.H. (Eds.) (1976). *The black church: A community resource for urban affairs and research.* Washington, DC: Howard University.

King, D.E. (1972). Worship in the black church. In E.L. McCall (Ed.), *The black Christian experience* (pp. 32-42). Nashville, TN: The Broadman Press.

Krause, N. (1992). Stress, religiosity, and psychological well-being among older blacks. *Journal of Aging and Health, 4*(3), 412-439.

Lincoln, C.E. (1995). Black religion and racial identity. In H.W. Harris, H.C. Blue, and E.H. Griffith (Eds.), *Racial and ethnic identity: Psychological development and creative expression* (pp. 209-221). New York: Routledge.

Lyles, M.R. (1992). Mental health perceptions of black pastors. Implications for psychotherapy with black patients. *Journal of Psychology and Christianity, 11*(4), 368-377.

McAdoo, H. and Crawford, V. (1991). The black church and family support programs. *Prevention in Human Services, 9*(1), 193-203.

Mitchell, H.H. (1972). Black preaching. In E.L. McCall (Ed.), *The black Christian experience* (pp. 43-62). Nashville, TN: The Broadman Press.

Morris, J.R. and Robinson, D.T. (1996). Community and Christianity in the black church. *Counseling and Values, 41*(1), 59-69.

Nye, W.P. (1992). Amazing grace: Religion and identity among elderly black individuals. *International Journal of Aging and Human Development, 36*(2), 103-114.

Payne, J.A. (Ed.) (1983). *Second Baptist Church 1863-1983.* Kansas City, MO: Second Baptist Church.

Pollard, W.L. (1978). *A study of black self-help.* San Francisco: R & E Research Associates.

Potts, R.G. (1996). Spirituality and the experience of cancer in an African-American community: Implications for psychosocial oncology. *Journal of Psychosocial Oncology, 14*(1), 1-19.

Ross, E.L. (Ed.) (1978). *Black heritage in social welfare 1860-1930.* Meluchen, NJ: Scarecrow Press.

Sanger, K.L. (1995). Slave resistance and rhetorical self-definition: Spirituals as a strategy. *Western Journal of Communication, 59*(3), 177-192.

Smith, J.M. (1993). Function and supportive roles of church and religion. In J.S. Jackson, L.M. Chatters, and R.J. Taylor (Eds.), *Aging in black America* (pp. 124-147). Newbury Park, CA: Sage Publications, Inc.

Sobel, M. (1988). *Trabelin' on: The slave journey to an Afro-Baptist faith.* Princeton, NJ: Princeton University Press.

Stewart, C.F. (1997). *Soul survivors: An African American spirituality.* Louisville, KY: Westminster John Knox Press.

Stillman, F.A., Bone, L.R., Rand, C., and Levine, D.M. (1993). Heart, body, and soul: A church-based smoking cessation program for urban African Americans. *Preventive Medicine, 22*(3), 335-349.

Sutherland, M., Hale, C.D., and Harris, G.J. (1995). Community health promotion: The church as partner. *Journal of Primary Prevention, 16*(2), 201-216.

Taylor, R.J. (1993). Religion and religious observances. In J.S. Jackson, L.M. Chatters, and R.J. Taylor (Eds.), *Aging in black America* (pp. 101-123). Newbury Park, CA: Sage Publications Inc.

Taylor, R.J. and Chatters, L.M. (1986). Patterns of informal support to elderly black adults: Family, friends, and church members. *Social Work, 31*(6), 432-438.

Taylor, R.J., Thornton, M.C., and Chatters, L.M. (1987). Black Americans' perceptions of the sociohistorical role of the church. *Journal of Black Studies, 18*(2), 123-138.

Thomas, S.T., Quinn, S.C., Billingsley, A., and Caldwell, C. (1994). The characteristics of northern black churches with community health outreach programs. *American Journal of Public Health, 84*(4), 575-579.

Thurman, H. (1975). *The Negro spiritual speaks of life and death.* Richmond, IN: Friends United Press.

Thurman, H. (1976). *Jesus and the disinherited.* Boston: Beacon Press.

Turner, L.W., Sutherland, M., Harris, G.J., and Barber, M. (1995). Cardiovascular health promotion in North Florida African-American churches. *Health Values: The Journal of Health Behavior, Education, and Promotion, 19*(2), 3-9.

Walker, W.T. (1976). The contemporary black church. In. D.J. Jones and W.H. Matthews (Eds.), *The black church: A community resource for urban affairs and research* (pp. 36-68). Washington, DC: Howard University.

Walls, C.T. (1992). The role of the church and family support in the lives of older African Americans. *Generations, 16*(3), 33-36.

Washington, J.M. (1994). *Conversations with God: Two centuries of prayers by African Americans.* New York: HarperCollins.

Westgate, C.E. (1996). Spiritual wellness and depression. *Journal of Counseling and Development, 75*(1), 26-35.

Wilson-Ford, V. (1992). Health-protective behaviors of rural black elderly women. *Health and Social Work, 17*(1), 28-35.

Wood, J.B. and Wan, T.T.H. (1993). Ethnicity and minority issues in family caregiving to rural black elders. In C.M. Barresi and D.E. Stull (Eds.), *Ethnic elderly and long-term care* (pp. 39-56). New York: Springer Publishing Company.

Wright, R. (1941). *12 million voices: A folk history of the Negro in the United States.* New York: Viking Press, p. 131.

Chapter 12

Augmenting Traditional Health Care Through Mutual Assistance Groups for Families

Edna Comer
Kathryn Kramer
Kermit B. Nash

INTRODUCTION

This chapter reports results of a study regarding twenty mutual assistance groups for parents of children with sickle-cell disease (SCD). Since groups for persons affected by SCD primarily serve African Americans, this information will help to increase awareness of the existence of mutual assistance groups serving this population. The chapter illustrates how the blending of traditional health care and mutual assistance groups can be an important resource for African-American families coping with chronic disease. In addition, it provides a foundation for discussion about the development of mutual assistance groups within the African-American community.

Traditionally, the health care system treats a person with a chronic illness as an individual with a medical problem. A more ecological perspective would examine the interrelatedness of the various aspects of a chronically ill person's life. Such factors as how the illness affects, and is affected by, immediate and extended families, the community, and society at large would be explored. From a family theory perspective, the support and information needed to cope with chronic illness may not always be readily available from within a medical setting. However, treatment intrinsically involves the family. As suggested in this chapter, psychosocial and social support needs of families are being addressed through a thirty-year-old movement called self-help (mutual assistance). While the common denominator of these groups is to help the family secure the well-being of the child, each group is different. Variation across groups presented in this study reflects the configuration of individual and environmental differences among communities. These findings support mutual help theory and research which suggests that focal problems and group and external environment interact to form a unique social niche within a community (Kramer and Nash, 1995; Maton, 1989).

This chapter addresses four areas: First, a framework for understanding mutual assistance groups, including a definition and brief history, is presented. Second, the rationale for advancing mutual assistance groups as a means of support for families affected by SCD is proposed. Third is a brief discussion regarding SCD and the manner in which it affects families. Fourth, methods used in this study are presented. Specific attention is given to activities and benefits reported by group members.

WHAT IS A MUTUAL ASSISTANCE GROUP?

The terms mutual assistance and/or mutual help are used frequently in the self-help literature (Kramer and Nash, 1995; Maton, 1989). A self-help or mutual support group may be conceptualized as the coming together of a small number of individuals encountering similar problems in health, mental health, or daily living. The purpose of the group is for giving and receiving help and support from one another (Borman, 1976; Kramer and Nash, 1995; Maton, 1989). Content used in these groups appears to be an overlap between self-help and support groups. Similar characteristics of mutual assistance and self-help groups include the notion of universality and acceptance and being a part of a group that understands the individual's experience (Borman, 1976). Professionals sometimes play a significant role in the founding and formation of these types of groups. On the other hand, mutual assistance groups such as support groups are member centered. Other commonalties between these two groups are that they are characterized by members sharing experiences, providing information, giving advice, and encouraging participation among themselves (Schopler and Galinsky, 1995).

History of Mutual Assistance Movement

In 1987, the Surgeon General of the United States, C. Everett Koop (1987), held a workshop on and organized a task force to examine the self-help and mutual assistance movement in this country. It was estimated that 500,000 mutual assistance groups serving 10 million people were active in the United States at that time. Current estimates vary from 6 million to 15 million people participating in mutual assistance groups across the United States. Although mutual assistance groups are composed of people with various needs, the purposes of all mutual assistance groups are the same: to provide emotional support to people who share the same predicament. Reissman and Gartner (1987) proposed that the ethos of mutual assistance is one of empowerment, self-determination, mutuality, noncommodity character of help, bottom-up orientation, and the integration of altruism and egoism.

Mutual assistance groups are abundant in this country and address almost every illness, disability, and life condition. The groups support individuals and help families cope by (1) providing education about the disease process and treatment, (2) informing about resources available, (3) providing emotional support, (4) offering a safe environment to express feelings and share interpersonal issues, and (5) in some cases, providing tangible resources.

Mutual Assistance Groups Benefit Families of Children with Chronic Illnesses

Self-help, support, or mutual assistance groups are recognized as an important part of the social support system for parents of children with chronic illnesses. Research has shown strong associations between a child's ability to cope with chronic illness and his or her parents' abilities to provide social support, open communication, understanding, and emotional and educational reinforcement to their children (Burlew, Evans, and Oler, 1989; Downe-Wamboldt and Ellerton, 1984; Monaco, 1988; Petr and Barney, 1993; Yoak, Chesney, and Schwartz, 1985). Parents' abilities to provide support for their children are often dependent on their obtaining support for themselves (Slaughter and Dilworth-Anderson, 1988).

Physiological symptomatology of a chronic illness strikes the child, and the child is the one who suffers from pain and degeneration of the body's cells, organs, and organ systems. However, it is argued that the treatment of children with chronic illnesses should be approached from a systems and social-ecological perspective (Kazak, 1986; Nebrig, 1991). When a child is being treated for a chronic illness, the child's family is his or her most important link for overall psychological support (Telfair, 1994). Evidence also suggests that the child's development is influenced indirectly by parental social networks (Cochran and Bassard, 1979).

Mutual assistance groups are recognized as an important part of the social support system for parents of children with cancer (Monaco, 1988), sickle-cell disease (Nash, 1990), and children with emotional and physical disabilities (Petr and Barney, 1993). Some of these parents report sharing a common bond that allows for understanding and support at the deepest level with other parents of children with similar illnesses. One study reported that parents realize myriad benefits from self-help groups (Downe-Wamboldt and Ellerton, 1984). Advantages gained from participation in the group include the following:

1. Acceptance of the abilities and limitations of the chronically ill child
2. Knowledge of the child's disease process and treatment
3. Assistance with parent-child issues such as discipline and fostering independence
4. Prevention of, and assistance in, crisis situations
5. Identification of strategies for normalizing family life and prevention of social isolation of family members
6. An opportunity to promote environmental and social change through a group process

One parent group of children with disabilities (physical and emotional) reported that the most reliable and inspirational source of support was other parents with children with similar disabilities (Petr and Barney, 1993). Perhaps most important are parents' reports of the benefits of self-help groups. One parent expressed the following sentiments:

> I think the people you meet are so incredible. Other parents—I think that's probably one of the biggest surprises to me. And I had friends before but somehow my friends who have kids with disabilities are so much more special to me. [They show] warmth [and] the ability to share very deep feelings at the drop of a hat. And you don't think twice about it because it's such a part of life. (Petr and Barney, 1993, p. 251)

Sickle-Cell Disease, Families, and Mutual Assistance Groups

Sickle-cell disease is a chronic illness, a genetic disorder that, in the United States, mainly affects African Americans. One in twelve African Americans carries the sickle-cell trait (Platt and Eckman, 1997; Weisman and Schechter, 1992). Sickle-cell anemia is found in about 1 of 400 births of African-American babies. Sickle-cell disease includes a group of blood disorders more specifically known as sickle-cell anemia hemoglobin with sickle abnormality. This condition causes severe pain in the joints and other parts of the body when red blood cells form rigid sickle-cell shapes. Among the complications of this disease are strokes, splenic involvement, enuresis, congestive heart failure, and renal failure.

Psychosocial complications for individuals with SCD and their families can contribute equally to difficulties in coping. Conyard, Krishnamurthy, and Doisk (1995) found that some parents of adolescents with this disease experience feelings of guilt. Burlew, Evans, and Oler (1989) suggest that SCD challenges the family on three levels: cognitively, emotionally, and behaviorally. Relative to cognition, the family is compelled to ascertain the course of the illness, etiology and prognosis, treatment options, and how the condition will affect the parent-child relationship. Emotional challenges to the family include being able to cope with "anxieties and uncertainties created by the illness" (p. 161). In addition, the family must determine how it will incorporate medical treatment needs of the child with daily living needs. Findings from a survey of 174 parents of children with SCD suggest that the disease imposes financial and emotional burdens on families (Whitten and Nishiura, 1985). For example, emergency medical care for children with SCD frequently requires that parents make arrangements for transportation, provide child care for other children in the home, and take days off work. In addition, parents reported being fearful and worried about their children's well-being.

Mutual assistance groups for SCD families have shown some benefits for parents from varied socioeconomic and educational backgrounds. One study reported that income levels of parents ranged from $1,400 to $45,000 annually (Nebrig, 1991). This same study showed that the level of education of parents in the group ranged from twelve to seventeen years. Other studies report that the participants are of varied racial/ethnic identities, including African Americans and Hispanic Americans (Nash, 1990; Nash and Kramer, 1993).

As a part of this trend, the number of mutual assistance groups for people with SCD is rapidly increasing in the United States. Since 1985, the number of known groups for people with SCD has more than doubled and is growing at an annual rate of 13.4 percent (Nash and Kramer, 1993). Findings from twenty groups of parents of children with SCD are presented in a later section.

METHODS

Through mail and telephone surveys, this project located twenty-four mutual assistance groups in the United States for parents of children with SCD. These groups were located in sixteen states and the District of Columbia. Of the twenty-four groups contacted, twenty agreed (83 percent) to participate in this study. Group leaders provided information on the structure and function of the groups.

Group leaders were contacted by phone to determine if their members would provide information on the members' experiences with the groups. Individual members from eleven of the twenty parent groups agreed to participate. These members represented groups in ten states. The leaders of these eleven groups estimated a total membership of 118 members. Questionnaires and consent forms were mailed to group leaders, and the leaders distributed the forms to members. Seventy-three members completed and returned individual questionnaires for a response rate of 62 percent.

Questionnaire Development

Questionnaire development was based on the recommendations of Dillman (1978) in *Mail and Telephone Survey: The Total Method*. Questionnaires used in this study were adapted from previous research projects in the Psychosocial Research Division of the Duke-UNC Comprehensive Sickle-Cell Center, Chapel Hill, North Carolina. The adapted versions were pilot tested at the University of North Carolina Hospital in the Sickle-Cell Clinic with parents of children with SCD.

RESULTS

Group-Level Data (Structural Variables)

The number of years groups had been in existence varied from zero to eighteen. The median number of years was four, and the mean was six. Group leaders reported that the groups met regularly, with 70 percent of the groups meeting twelve times a year or an average of once a month.

An average of twelve individuals regularly attended the parent self-help groups meetings. Of regular attendees, there were three times as many women attending as men. Children attended 30 percent of the groups but did not participate in the group's activities or discussions.

Demographics of Individual Members (Parents)

Considerable variability in the ages of the participants was noted, with a range of twelve to seventy-five years. The younger ages represented children who attended but did not participate in the groups. The median age of participants was thirty-six years, and the mean was thirty-seven. Of the participants, 97 percent were African

Americans, 90 percent were female, 10 percent were male, and 61 percent were single parents. Forty-two percent had completed high school, 37 percent had some college or technical training, 10 percent completed college, and 6 percent had some graduate training. Fifty-six percent were employed, 20 percent identified themselves as homemakers, and 63 percent reported annual incomes less than $25,000.

Group Activities

Group leaders were asked to report how often members of the groups participated in specific activities, such as talk about things that cause stress for the family or prayer during the meeting. Based on responses, groups appeared to be engaging in multiple activities or processes, such as providing education, emotional support, and advocacy for their members. Multiple activities conducted within groups suggest that typology by group process varies depending on the specific needs of the group. Although groups reported a wide variety of activities, four activities occurred most often:

1. Give advice to one another (95 percent, sometimes or very often)
2. Talk about things that cause stress on the family (95 percent, sometimes or very often)
3. Listen to experts discuss SCD (95 percent, sometimes or very often)
4. Talk about very personal feelings (90 percent, sometimes or very often) (see Table 12.1)

Special Features of Groups

This study found that 50 percent of the groups were led by a member of the group, 25 percent of the groups were led by a professional, and 10 percent were co-led by a professional and a group member. Of the groups, 15 percent did not report group leadership.

TABLE 12.1. Group Activities (n = 20)

Activity	Never %	Almost Never %	Some-times %	Very Often %
Talk about things that cause stress on the family	0	5	25	70
Talk about very personal things	0	10	60	30
Talk about recent advances in treatment	0	30	35	25
Learn how to deal with certain situations	10	30	35	25
Practice dealing with certain situations	55	20	15	10
Give advice to one another	0	5	10	85
Plan to change things in the hospital clinic	15	25	50	10
Plan to get together socially	15	10	55	20
Talk about how to recruit new members	5	15	20	60
Pray	35	5	10	50
Listen to experts discuss SCD	0	5	58	37

Group leaders were asked to identify special features of their groups. The most frequently stated features were that the group helped to provide transportation for hospital visits (75 percent) and pushed for change in social and/or health policies (73 percent). Other features provided by 50 percent or more of the groups were providing transportation to meetings, offering a buddy system, and having speakers (from the group) present for other groups (see Table 12.2).

Reasons for Group Participation

Parents reported several reasons for participation in the groups. Rationales for attending groups may be categorized in three areas. First, 87 percent of participants indicated their attendance was motivated by the desire to learn more about SCD and to improve health care for people with SCD. Second, 78 percent and 79 percent, respectively, reported that they attended to be supportive and to receive support. Last, over 50 percent of participants reported other reasons for attending, including to become more skillful at problem solving, raise money for SCD-related problems, and have a safe place to express feelings (see Table 12.3).

TABLE 12.2. Special Features of Parent Mutual Assistance Groups (n = 20)

Greater Than 50 Percent of All Parent Groups	
Special Features	**Percent**
Hospital visits	75
Advocate for changes	73
Transportation to meetings	60
Buddy system	50
Speakers for other groups	50
Less Than 50 Percent of All Parent Groups	
Contribute funds to needy members	45
Baby-sitting during meetings	45
Transportation to appointments	45
Home visits	35
Newsletter	25
Baby-sitting/respite care	25
Raise funds for hospital or clinic	20

Benefits from Group Participation

Every participant reported getting some benefit from group participation (see Table 12.4). Over 50 percent of the participants reported receiving the most benefit in the following areas:

1. Getting information about SCD (77 percent)
2. Getting advice/support from others (62 percent)
3. Feeling free to express feelings (60 percent)
4. Expressing compassion or care for others (60 percent)
5. Meeting others with similar problems (56 percent)
6 Coping with attitudes toward child's illness (51 percent)
7. Becoming more helpful (51 percent)

TABLE 12.3. Individuals' Reasons for Attending (n = 77)

Reason	Percent Responding "Yes"
To learn more about SCD	87
To improve health care for people with SCD	87
To give support	79
To get support	78
To learn how to solve personal problems	53
To raise money for causes	53
To have a safe place to express feelings	51
To make new friends	48
To have social activities	39
To have a sense of belonging to a group	33

TABLE 12.4. Benefits from Group Participation

Benefit	% Receiving Much Benefit
Information regarding SCD	77
Getting advice/support from others	62
Feeling free to express feelings	60
Expressing and learning compassion or care for others*	60
Meeting others with similar problems	56
Coping with attitudes toward child's illness	51
Becoming more helpful	51
Getting help from others	44
Learning how to deal with problems by watching others	42
Being helpful to others	41
Learning one's rights as an individual	40
Feeling part of a larger group	38
Being supported, approved of	36
Coping with problems in the family	35
Learning to cope differently	35
Developing self-confidence	35
Learning how to be a leader	33
Feeling spiritually uplifted	32
Having more fun	30
Changing things in the hospital	17

Note: Rank ordered from most highly endorsed to least.
*Everyone answering the questionnaire reported some benefit in this area.

SUMMARY

The twenty groups in this study were made up of individuals of different ages and educational and socioeconomic levels. These groups were located in different communities, each with its own ecological uniqueness. Nevertheless, most participants in this study realized some benefits from taking part in these groups. For example, parents reported giving advice and sharing personal feelings about SCD, hearing others' experiences with SCD, and discussing ways in which SCD affects families. These activities provided an opportunity for parents of children with SCD to interact and develop a relationship with other parents with similar experiences and concerns. Parents also obtained information from experts about issues related to SCD. In addition, being a member of a group appears to have resulted in special gains for some parents, including transportation to medical appointments, providing others with information about SCD, and support in advocating for change in social and health policies.

CONCLUSION

This study provides the first data on groups primarily serving African-American families and, thus, is an important contribution to the literature. Since no prior data existed, it was critical to begin discovering the location and structure of the groups. Equally important was gathering data regarding activities and special features of groups, the characteristics of group members and leaders, the reasons persons chose to attend, and the benefits they perceived from attending. Although methodological limitations are associated with qualitative, descriptive studies (e.g., external validity issues), it is hoped that this study will lay the foundation for future research in this area that is more rigorous.

From a family perspective, the support and information needed to cope with chronic illness may not always be readily available from within a medical setting. In response, individuals are turning to one another for social support through mutual assistance groups. These groups provide a variety of functions, including education, support, and social activities. In addition, many groups help advocate for persons affected by chronic illness, and some groups are actively involved in health care reform. The prevalence of mutual assistance groups is noteworthy because such groups are clearly meeting individual needs and augmenting the traditional health care delivery system.

REFERENCES

Borman, L. (1976). Self-help and the professional. *Social Policy, 7*(1), 46-47.

Burlew, D., Evans, R., and Oler, C. (1989). The impact of a child with sickle cell disease on family dynamics. *Annals New York Academy of Science, 56*(5), 161-171.

Cochran, M. and Bassard, J. (1979). Child development and personal social networks. *Child Development, 50*(3), 601-616.

Conyard, S., Krishnamurthy, M., and Doisk, H. (1995). Psychosocial aspects of sickle cell anemia in adolescents. In F.J. Turner (Ed.), *Differential diagnosis and treatment* (pp. 286-294). New York: The Free Press.

Dillman, D. (1978). *Mail and telephone survey: The total method.* New York: John Wiley and Sons.

Downe-Wamboldt, B. and Ellerton, M. (1984). The parent connection: Self-help for families of chronically ill children. *The Australian Nurses Journal, 13*(11), 50-52.

Kazak, A.E. (1986). Families with physically handicapped children: Social ecology and family systems. *Family Process, 25*(2), 265-281.

Koop, C. (1987). *The surgeon general's workshop on self-help and public health.* Los Angeles, CA: U.S. Department of Health and Human Resources. September 20-22.

Kramer, K.D. and Nash, K.B. (1995). The unique ecology of groups: Findings from groups for African Americans affected by sickle-cell disease. In M. Galinsky and J. Schopler (Eds.), *Support groups: Current perspectives on theory and practice* (pp. 55-65). Binghamton, NY: The Haworth Press, Inc.

Maton, K.I. (1989). Toward an ecological understanding of mutual-help groups: The social ecology of "fit." *American Journal of Community Psychology, 17*(6), 729-753.

Monaco, G. (1988). Parent self-help groups for families of children with cancer. *CA-A Cancer Journal for Clinicians, 38*(3), 169-174.

Nash, K.B. (1990). *A psychosocial perspective: Growing up with thalassemia, a chronic disorder.* Paper presented at the Sixth Cooley's Anemia Symposium, The New York Academy of Sciences, New York, New York Sheraton Center Hotel, March 6-8.

Nash, K. and Kramer, K. (1993). Self-help for sickle cell disease in African American communities. *The Journal of Applied Behavioral Science, 29*(2), 202-215.

Nebrig, D.E. (1991). Self-help groups for parents of children with sickle cell disease: A comparison of the characteristics of groups, group leaders, and parent members. Unpublished master's thesis, Chapel Hill, NC: University of North Carolina School of Social Work.

Petr, C.G. and Barney, D. (1993). Reasonable efforts for children with disabilities: The parents' perspective. *Journal of Social Work, 38*(3), 247-254.

Platt, A. and Eckman, W. (1997). Grappling with sickle cell: Diagnosing and managing hemoglobin disorders. *Advance for Physician Assistants, 1*(2), 21-24.

Reissman, F. and Gartner, A. (1987). The surgeon general and the self-help ethos. *Social Policy, 1*(2), Fall, 23-25.

Schopler, J.H. and Galinsky, M.J. (1995). Expanding our view of support groups as an open system. In M. Galinsky and J. Schopler (Eds.), *Support groups: Current perspectives on theory and practice* (pp. 3-10). Binghamton, NY: The Haworth Press, Inc.

Slaughter, B. and Dilworth-Anderson, P. (1988). Care of black children with sickle cell disease: Fathers, maternal support, and esteem. *Family Relations, 37*(3), 281-287.

Telfair, J. (1994). Factors in the long term adjustment of children and adolescents with sickle cell disease: Conceptualizations and review of literature. *Health and Social Policy, 5*(3/4), 69-96.

Weisman, S.J. and Schechter, N.L. (1992). Sickle cell anemia: Pain management. In R.S. Sinatra, A. Hord, B. Ginsberg, and L. Preble (Eds.), *Acute pain: Mechanisms and management* (pp. 508-516). New York: Mosby Yearbook.

Whitten, C.F. and Nishiura, E.N. (1985). Sickle cell anemia. In N. Hobbs and J. Perrin (Eds.), *Issues in the care of children with chronic illness* (pp. 236-260). San Franciso: Jossey-Bass Publishers.

Yoak, M., Chesney, B., and Schwartz, N. (1985). Active roles in self-help groups for parents of children with cancer. *Children's Health Care, 14*(1), 38-45.

Chapter 13

African-Centered Community Building: Implications for Political Action and Systems Change

Edith M. Freeman

Traditional health concepts are inadequate for furthering our understanding of life in black communities for a number of reasons. Most of those concepts have been derived from the medical model. That model is too linear in its focus; consequently, it fails to consider the rich, multilayered nature of life in those communities, which is influenced by many interacting factors. Use of the medical model limits the focus to individual factors in isolation of the environmental context, encouraging a blaming of the person. Stereotyping and blaming have led to an emphasis on pathology rather than strengths, (Weick, 1985) and may have encouraged a proliferation of culturally biased, negatively focused research on black communities.

Community practice approaches have been proposed as an alternative to such culturally biased perspectives. Community approaches provide guidelines for exploring the cultural environments of all families, and for organizing and implementing health promotion strategies. Philosophically, community practice approaches are more consistent with the strengths, social justice, and empowerment orientation of social work than individually focused approaches (Gutierrez et al., 1996; Saleebey, 1996; Solomon, 1987). Moreover, these approaches can be more culturally relevant to black families and communities because they help practitioners, policymakers, and researchers to explore cultural resources and supports, as well as institutional and individual barriers to self- and collective sufficiency.

This chapter summarizes some of the practice approaches currently used within communities, and identifies which of those approaches are more responsive to black families' needs, to a health promotion philosophy, and to systems changes. The full-partnership or community-building approach is then discussed as a core component of an African-centered framework for health promotion and capacity building. An example of community building illustrates how this African-centered approach works and the strengths orientation it requires for community practitioners and service providers. Finally, the implications for future practice with this approach are discussed.

COMMUNITY PRACTICE APPROACHES AND HEALTH PROMOTION

Health Promotion's Philosophical Underpinnings

The recent trend has been toward comprehensive approaches to health promotion that build on a community's capacity to support its members' healthy lifestyles. An underlying philosophy emphasizes that a community's health is not only related to its health care resources but also to other factors, such as its economic, social, cultural, and political strengths and barriers. Health promotion, in contrast to traditional health approaches, is focused on enhancing and preserving health rather than on simply treating illnesses (Caplan et al., 1989). The emphasis is also on primary and secondary prevention and on services integration. Hence, these comprehensive approaches require the integration of a range of human services, including health, education, housing, employment, mental health, legal, aging, and child welfare services. The goal is increased accessibility of services by encouraging community members to become actively involved in designing and implementing culturally relevant services and policies.

Comprehensive approaches are especially important in impoverished communities and in communities of color. In those communities, formal resources may be more limited than in affluent communities, and the residents' strengths and resiliency may be ignored by those in power. In some black communities, for example, biased legislative funding may provide only health maintenance and emergency services, without including health promotion programs. Mutual help and other cultural supports might be used to supplement these formal services, but they are often insufficient for resolving long-standing systemic risk conditions. Moreover, some health promotion and social programs in black communities, in spite of an empowerment philosophy, may not involve input from those communities about their unique needs, cultural strengths, and culturally relevant services. Such programs may ignore environmental barriers, such as inadequate employment and housing resources or lack of opportunity to influence decision makers, that can impact upon a community's health.

One example involves a statewide substance abuse prevention and health promotion program with an empowerment and community-centered philosophy. Parents in each community were asked to provide feedback about a generic parent effectiveness curriculum that was being considered as part of the program. When black and Latino communities across the state requested that culture-specific parenting programs be adopted for their communities as an alternative, they were told that such programs did not exist, although they had provided the names of relevant programs with their requests. Evaluations of the generic program over the next two years yielded consistent feedback from these communities about a lack of respect for their input and the cultural biases implicit in the program that was adopted by the state. The stress and frustration from this experience with environmental barriers probably impacted negatively upon the physical and mental health of these community residents.

As can be seen from this example, respect for community input is an essential aspect of a health promotion philosophy. Such a philosophy helps to achieve the empowerment goals of comprehensive community practice approaches. Although community professionals have expertise in many key areas, it is assumed that residents are experts regarding their community experiences and ability to identify culturally relevant program components that can meet their needs. Briar-Lawson and colleagues (1997) categorized a range of school-linked community programs and approaches into first- and second-generation approaches. These categories are based on each approach's philosophy about the balance between community residents' and professionals' input into program planning, implementation, and evaluation.

First-Generation Approaches

Figure 13.1 includes a range of community practice approaches to health promotion. First-generation approaches, according to Briar-Lawson and colleagues (1997), emphasize colocation of services and services integration. Such services tend to be child, organization, or professional discipline centered. In Table 13.1, exam-

FIGURE 13.1. An Afrocentric Community-Building Framework

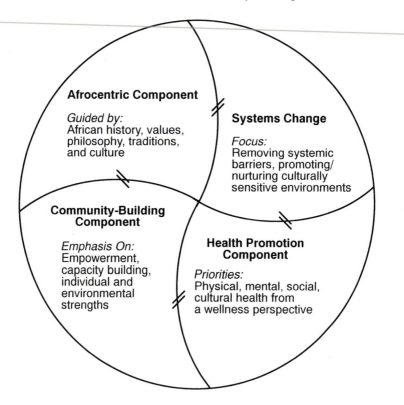

Key: // = Areas of interchange and integration between components.

TABLE 13.1. Community Practice Approach to Health Promotion

First-Generation Programs		Second-Generation Programs	
Coordination Approach	**Consultation Approach**	**Collaboration Approach**	**Full-Partnership/ Community-Building Approach**
Organization and child centered	Professional discipline centered	Family centered	Family and community centered
No input from community residents	Little input from community residents	Involvement of indigenous leaders and organizations	Total agenda set by the community residents, networks, and leaders
Key stakeholders are service-providing organizations and professionals	Key stakeholders are selected individuals at the decision-making table, generally professionals	Key stakeholders include select segments of the community and professionals	Key stakeholders include all who have an interest in and are concerned about community issues
Coordinator and educator roles	Intervenor, consultant, and educator roles	Interprofessional team leader or member, collaborator, advocate, educator roles	Facilitator, catalyst, coach, advocate, educator, learner roles
Outcomes			
Improved service network in communities regarding fragmentation and accountability	Agenda set by experts internal or external to community	Agenda set by collaborative team	Coalition leadership development, capacity building
Network agenda setting	Improved problem-solving skills by providers	Individual and family change, system change is coincidental	Individual and family change, and planned systems change

ples of first-generation programs use the approaches of coordination and consultation. The amount of input from community members ranges from little to no input into decision making. Partnership opportunities within first-generation programs exist between professionals only, based on their assumed expertise. Thus, power-sharing activities tend to exclude families and other community members (Kirst, 1996; Melaville and Blank, 1993).

One example of a first-generation approach involves a private foundation that developed a comprehensive early childhood, child-centered, education and health promotion program. The program shifted its focus to include community empowerment and development, as staff began to encounter numerous environmental barriers. The community was triethnic, including African-American, Latino, and white members. The main point of entry for the program was expected to be a primarily Latino community health clinic. Expert consultants and interagency partners or networks of professionals had been involved in planning, coordinating, and implementing the program at various phases of its development.

Then, community input was solicited through several community forums in which residents were asked to react to the fully developed plan. Feedback indicated that few African-American families used the designated health clinic because they felt unwelcome and disrespected by the staff, so they chose to use a health clinic outside their community. The planning group decided not to include African-American families in the program because they assumed that health, and by implication health promotion, was not a priority for those families. In this example of a first-generation program, the community members were not included as partners in the initial phases of planning and implementing the program. Moreover, even when their input was solicited after the program was developed, their expert knowledge about their experiences with the health clinic and other aspects of the community was viewed through the professionals' value biases. Consequently, opportunities for capacity building, for enhancing and developing the African-American families' leadership and health promotion skills, were lost.

Second-Generation Approaches

Table 13.1 also reflects important characteristics of second-generation community approaches in relation to health promotion, including family and/or community centeredness. Examples of such approaches include family-centered collaboration and the full-partnership/community-building approaches. "In second-generation partnerships, families and community members are joint leaders" (Briar-Lawson et al., 1997, p. 142), along with community professionals. In the collaborative approach, interprofessional teams that include families and community members set the agenda, whereas in the community-building approach, the agenda is set by the community, with professionals facilitating the process.

With second-generation approaches, families and community members are invited to the planning and decision-making table during initial discussions. Such discussions should precede the conducting of needs and strengths assessments, such as assets mapping, to engage communities in the process of deciding how their needs and goals will be explored and discovered. Second-generation approaches assume that this initial time investment is often required for trust and relationship building, consistent with cultural expectations among African Americans, Latinos, and other communities of color. Moreover, the capacity-building aspects of these approaches involve helping communities to identify opportunities to develop, enhance, and practice their leadership and political action skills.

The empowerment and strengths-oriented focus of second-generation approaches implies that such opportunities and skills often exist in communities prior to professional intervention. The residents' cultural priorities, rather than professional agendas, should determine how this capacity-enhancing and capacity-building process unfolds (Briar-Lawson et al., 1997). Poole (1995, p. 1158) concurs regarding the goal of these approaches: "They seek to enhance and preserve the physical, mental, and social health of clients as well as families, neighborhoods, and other natural support systems."

One comprehensive health center decided to develop a community-centered health promotion initiative in a predominantly African-American community. The planners needed to enlist the community's support for a grant application for HIV/AIDS, teen pregnancy, and childhood asthma prevention. The grant required a full-partnership/community-building approach, similar to Briar-Lawson and colleagues' (1997) second-generation programs. The planners used a key informant approach to identify natural leaders and networks within the community, as well as settings where residents could be contacted informally, such as political and social clubs, small restaurants, barber and beauty shops, lodges, and churches. During several weeks of discussions with residents about their concerns, the issue of transportation surfaced many times.

City bus service was provided only in the community's outer perimeters and was limited to morning and evening rush hours. Many residents did not own cars, so getting to work and to other appointments was difficult for them. The health center planners agreed that transportation seemed to be a community priority, and that the bus company's previous routing decisions might be discriminatory, but they reminded the residents that their focus was on health. The residents linked their frustration and stress about the transportation problem to their mental health and to the planners' initial promise to respond to the community's concerns.

Therefore, the planners decided to help the residents organize a letter-writing campaign and a face-to-face meeting with the bus company. The company agreed to provide two new routes within the community on a thirty-day trial basis to determine if there was sufficient demand for the service. The residents then organized their own bus-riding campaign, which included enlisting other residents who owned cars to park their cars and ride the buses. The campaign was successful. This initial partnership between the community and the health center planners became the foundation for the subsequent grant application and program development phases of the project. The experience utilized some residents' existing political action skills and helped others to develop those skills. The power sharing between professionals and residents also increased the latter's self- and collective efficacy. Furthermore, the experience allowed the planners to operationalize their empowerment and health promotion philosophy, and allowed the community to set its own agenda, as expected in second-generation community-building programs.

AN AFRICAN-CENTERED COMMUNITY-BUILDING FRAMEWORK

Overview of the Framework

The movement toward second-generation programs and approaches highlights many lessons that have been learned. One important lesson is the need for cultural sensitivity regarding the strengths and oppression experiences of people of color. The literature is just beginning to address how cultural sensitivity and, more important, cultural competence can be achieved by practitioners, administrators, and policymakers. A number of approaches have been identified to help community professionals achieve this goal. The following discussion clarifies how some of these approaches, in combination, can be organized as a framework for community building and health promotion in African-American communities.

Core Components of the Framework

The core components of this framework include African values and philosophy, health promotion, community building, and systems change. Figure 13.1 illustrates the dynamic interrelationships between these components as well as the essential aspects they contribute to the framework. These components are discussed separately for clarity, but they can only be understood in terms of their reciprocal influences on one another, as they are implemented in black communities. This framework requires the development of full partnerships between African-American families and community members, community practitioners, funders, policymakers, researchers, and service providers.

The Afrocentric Component

Afrocentricity has been defined as "the internalization of values that emphasize love of self, awareness of one's traditional African cultural heritage, and personal commitment to the economic/political development of African Americans and other people of African descent" (Oliver, 1989, p. 26). It is both a way of life and an intervention paradigm (Crawley and Freeman, 1993). As an intervention paradigm, the concept implies that the cultural values of African Americans should be used as the theoretical base for developing culturally relevant practice approaches. Schiele (1996, p. 284) notes that to do less implies that "Eurocentric values are the only values that can explain behavior and should be the basis for solving peoples' problems." (See Chapter 8 as an example of African-centered intervention with families.)

In contrast to Eurocentric values, the Afrocentric paradigm is guided by the following value assumptions: (1) human identity is a collective identity, (2) the spiritual or nonmaterial component of human beings is just as important as the material component, and

(3) the affective approach to knowledge is epistemologically valid (Akbar, 1984; Asante, 1988; Harris, 1992; Nobles, 1980; Schiele, 1990). Although individual uniqueness is acknowledged, it is assumed that the individual cannot be understood separately from his or her cultural or social group. In traditional African philosophy, all human beings are viewed as connected to one another, to nature, and to a Supreme Being, while soul, mind, and body are considered interdependent and interrelated. The paradigm asserts that feelings and emotions are a valid and valued source of knowing, and that they are the most direct expression of self. Rationality and emotionality are viewed as two sides of the same coin, as a union of opposites, or how people experience life holistically (Akbar, 1984; Nobles, 1980; Schiele, 1994).

Hence, Afrocentricity provides a set of values, a philosophy, and a combination of culturally centered interventions that can improve the cultural relevance of health promotion efforts in African-American communities. Table 13.2 includes examples of interventions that help such communities create an Afrocentric milieu for families and other residents. As can be seen from this table, those interventions range from how those families are to be in the world (group identity), to knowing (the joining of emotionality and rationality), to centering (spiritual, natural, and relational connections), to creating (contributing to current and future generations).

These interventions are relevant to the cultural values and traditions of African Americans. For example, oral histories and narratives help center African-American communities by codifying their positive coping experiences and resiliencies, as well as successful efforts to change discriminatory policies and practices. Those narratives can also be used to socialize youths in mentoring circles, which are an African tradition, to honor elders, and to create new leadership among the young. These interventions are discussed in more detail in the community-building example in a later section.

The Health Promotion Component

As the second component of this African-centered framework, health promotion, which was discussed in a previous section, includes a broader definition of health. First, in this framework,

TABLE 13.2. Services and Interventions Useful for Helping Communities to Develop an Afrocentric Milieu

Afrocentric Philosophy and Values	Examples of Cultural Rituals and Traditions (Services and Interventions)
Ways of being in the world; maintaining connections (group identity)	• Naming ceremonies • Kwanza celebrations • Life in extended family clans, tribes, and social networks
Knowing (integration of emotionality and rationality and equals holistic)	• Inductive learning styles • African drumming, singing, and dancing ceremonies • Healing rituals
Centering (spirituality, eldership, balance between self and nature, emphasis on relationships)	• Oral histories and heritage books • Fasting and cleansing rituals
Creating and preserving (influencing current and future generations)	• Mentoring circles • Rites of passage • Service to community/clan • Political and economic development for African-descended people

physical and mental health are viewed on a single continuum, with a large overlap area near the midpoint of the continuum. Each area of health is assumed to be heavily influenced by and to influence the other; consequently, it is extremely difficult to separate these two aspects of health. Another assumption is that environmental barriers and racial and ethnic stress, as well as cultural strengths, affect the physical and mental health of African-American communities. For example, a black person's prognosis related to diseases such as diabetes and high blood pressure is directly affected by biological factors, mental health, physical health, and other socially and culturally determined factors. The prognosis may be affected by the individual's family history, cultural dietary patterns, access to resources for adequate nutrition education and nutrition, and psychological coping. Hence, to be effective, this health promotion and community-building component addresses this important connection.

Second, a community's sociocultural health should be assessed in terms of its coping responses to the adverse social and racial stress confronted by its members (Hardy-Fanta, 1986). The concept of sociocultural health directs attention to the resiliency and strengths of African-American communities that have helped them to survive adverse conditions and, in many instances, to thrive in spite of those conditions.

For example, research has documented that the rates of mental illness are roughly the same across all racial/ethnic groups and countries (Read, 1992), although African Americans and other people of color are more likely to be labeled with certain diagnoses, such as schizophrenia, than others (Read, 1992). This finding indicates that African-American communities are extremely resilient in coping with the social, political, and cultural barriers in their environments. Sociocultural health is, therefore, a more culturally relevant concept related to black communities than physical or mental health alone. Sociocultural health makes this framework much more relevant to black communities and to their unique combination of strengths and needs.

Systems Change Component

While assessing and supporting coping and resiliency in African-American communities is an important aspect of this framework, systems change is an essential third component (see Figure 13.1). Hence, the framework is designed to strengthen both coping and problem-solving resources of community residents and their environmental resources. For example, providing educational sessions to help residents in impoverished communities to learn small business development skills is insufficient by itself (Burwell, 1995). Those economic development activities should be accompanied by political action and advocacy to reform discriminatory bank financing policies and to build coalitions with established business leaders for mentoring, training, and networking purposes.

The goal of this component is mobilization and coalition building, political action, advocacy, economic development, local services development, and, most important, institutional and policy reform (Checkoway, 1995; Gutierrez and Lewis, 1994; Raheim and Bolden, 1995; Weil and Gamble, 1995). In this component, and in the framework as a whole, the choice of strategy, method of use, the stakeholders to be involved, and the timing should be determined by the cultural and value priorities of the community residents.

The Community-Building Component

The community-building approach described in a previous section on community building and health promotion is a fourth component of this framework. The goal of this component is community education, citizen participation and leadership development, and economic and political development (Checkoway, 1995; Cox, 1991). The use of these strategies should help African-American communities enhance their existing infrastructure and develop missing areas of infrastructure. The emphasis is not only on capacity building through an improved infrastructure (viable leadership, networks, organizational and community structure) but also through improved abilities and skills of individual residents.

Cultural traditions should determine the nature of that structure; for example, the black church is one organizational, political, and economic structure that functions differently than the infrastructure in other communities. In efforts to help African-American communities with community building, it is a mistake to view the black church only as a religious institution. In fact, Weil and Gamble (1995, p. 578) indicate that "many support and aid groups and community development projects have been formed through the African-American church" (see Chapter 11 for further elaboration of this example). It is also important to acknowledge spiritual values and organizational dynamics that are part of this infrastructure. For instance, health promotion and community-building programs in black churches, such as HIV/AIDS, substance abuse, or pregnancy prevention, may encounter political, class, or economic as well as religious barriers. As can be seen from Figure 13.1, and from this discussion, there is much overlap and synergy among the four components of this framework.

AN AFROCENTRIC COMMUNITY-BUILDING HEALTH PROMOTION EXAMPLE

Although a number of communities are using aspects of the framework from the previous section in combination with other approaches, few of them are using all four components. Use of this framework is consistent with the current trend toward combining economic and social development approaches in community practice (Weil, 1996). In the following community example, the value of these development approaches is evident in the capacity-building process that occurred.

Project Overview and Mission

The Zion Grove Baptist Housing Development is a church-sponsored inner-city housing complex that was established for elderly African-American residents in the early 1980s. However, the planners overestimated the need for senior housing in this West Coast community. Therefore, after several years of low occupancy, the policy was changed to allow families with children to move into the development. This change created a need for policy reforms in other areas, and, eventually, a tenants' association developed among the residents to address the ongoing needs. Then, as other broader community issues emerged, such as violence, drug abuse, school dropouts, unemployment and inadequate economic development, and lack of recreation resources, it became apparent that the housing development and surrounding community had many mutual concerns. The tenants' association developed a coalition with other parts of the community that eventually included a hospital, a community action group, a community center, two churches, a high school, and an elementary magnet (specialized and student-centered) school with an Afrocentric curriculum.

Over a ten-year period, by applying for funding from diverse sources and hiring staff as well as indigenous leaders, the project has developed a range of integrated and comprehensive services. Funders include federal and state housing, public health, substance abuse prevention, criminal justice, and agriculture departments, as well as private funding for community-centered initiatives. Gradually, the project has evolved into a second-generation community-building program. The range of services include many that fall within the four components of the African-centered framework discussed in the previous section, along with other services. The services are coordinated by a central board that represents all of the coalition's partners, including families and other community members who were involved in the initial coalition-building and planning phase. This combination of services is guided by the project's mission: to enhance the community's power to make major decisions that affect its well-being, and to increase its collective sufficiency through a process of community-building and empowerment.

The Four Core Components

The Afrocentric Component

The schools and the community center are the lead agencies for this component, which extends the elementary magnet school's Afrocentric curriculum into the community. The component includes a community education program on African and African-American history and traditions for individuals, families, and groups. This component uses the village concept to encourage all adults to exercise their responsibility for contributing to current and future generations by mentoring and supporting children and youths. Separate male and female circles, based on an African tradition, are used to help seniors to mentor and socialize youths in culturally meaningful ways.

Rites of passage are also used to ritualize youths' movement into the older teenage and young adult years through cultural education, community service projects, and new family roles. Youths and adults can participate in African drumming, singing, spirituality, and dancing classes, as well as discussion groups focused on African and African-American art, films, and literature. The Afrocentric component also helps to shape the services provided through the other three components.

Health Promotion Component

Health promotion builds on the Afrocentric component; for instance, services include an intergenerational mentoring project focused on seniors teaching youths flower, herb, and vegetable gardening. Seniors structure the work and interactions to teach the youths discipline, community responsibility, and problem solving.

The vegetable and herb gardens include teaching about African traditions around communal farming, cooking, and healing. The flower and landscape gardening is part of a community beautification project in which the youths and seniors provide flora to improve areas surrounding the housing development and other key sites in the community. Often, youths who have been "jumped out" of gangs, or beaten severely by gang members for wanting to leave, begin their rebirth as nongang members by participating in the beautification project.

The health component also includes a wellness and community education program focused on nutrition, exercise, stress reduction, and health self-assessments; an HIV/AIDS prevention program; and a substance abuse prevention and early intervention program that targets youths, seniors, and single mothers as high-risk groups. The nutrition and stress reduction services address traditional and healthy aspects of African and African-American diet and cooking. These services focus on the effects of racial oppression and discrimination on stress, and the importance of culturally adaptive coping styles. Among the coalition's members, the church and hospital primarily coordinate the health promotion component. The church has always had an urban mission that includes a well-baby clinic and consumer education classes, while the hospital recently established a community-centered initiative as one of its new priorities.

The Community-Building and Systems Changes Components

Through the process of planning and implementation, the community has found that these two components are closely integrated and difficult to separate. The community-building component has a consumer education program and a gang prevention program. The latter includes family education and support, along with direct services to youths. This component is responsible for periodic strengths and needs assessments of the community, or assets mapping, for census, voter redistricting, and marketing/economic development purposes. Another part of this component is a community and economic development program that helps residents secure loans for housing and for starting or maintaining businesses. This program also establishes economic development projects, such as a housing development and a trash collection business. The trash business hires community residents and involves a large number of community volunteers.

Related to the economic development area, the systems changes component includes a leadership development and entrepreneurial project that pairs community residents with business leaders. The focus is on providing the residents with mentoring, support, career guidance, and information about starting small businesses or finding employment opportunities. Hence, the project's philosophy of both community building and systems changes, or enhancing internal and external resources, is expressed in the linkage between these two components. The landlord-tenant services, mediation and housing policy reforms and implementation, along with welfare-to-work, or the Temporary Assistance to Needy Families (TANF) program and policy reforms, are also part of the systems changes component. One important accomplishment of the project has been the coalition's effective advocacy for getting TANF participants involved in the Afrocentric cultural education classes and wellness program. The coalition believed that those classes were essential for the participants' successful entry into the world of work, by helping to increase their self- and cultural esteem and health promotion knowledge and skills.

IMPLICATIONS FOR FUTURE PRACTICE WITH THIS FRAMEWORK

The previous community-building health promotion example illustrates some of the complexities in implementing these strategies in African-American communities. In addition, other implications include residents' and service providers' value conflicts concerning cultural identity and health promotion strategies, the need for further framework model development, and research and evaluation issues.

Implementation Difficulties

Implementing comprehensive second-generation community-building programs can be difficult for a number of reasons. The emphasis on families and other community residents as full partners is a valuable philosophical tenet. However, in the Zion Grove project, and others, service providers continually struggle with how to support a community agenda with which they do not agree, or that they believe will be ineffective. They struggle too with how to help community residents maintain a balance between direct services designed to help individuals and families and those targeted toward systems changes (Freeman and O'Dell, 1997). The framework's guidelines emphasize change at the micro, mezzo, and macro levels. In many ways, macro change is more difficult, and some African-American communities may be overwhelmed and hopeless about their ability to influence large systems changes. Clearly, the process of involving all partners in grappling with and resolving these implementation difficulties is as important as the outcomes.

Value Conflicts

Value conflicts may develop not only between service providers and residents but also among residents (Weil and Gamble, 1995). In many African-American communities, socioeconomic class, regional, and international differences exist. For example, value and lifestyle differences may exist between poor residents and those with middle incomes, between residents from the rural South and those from urban areas on the East Coast, and between those born in America and those born in the Caribbean. Such differences often influence how residents define their needs and strengths, their value priorities, their partnership roles, and the services they desire.

Hence, differences among community residents can affect whether consensus develops and how providers facilitate or help residents manage those differences. In the Zion Grove project, for instance, political and class differences led to conflicts over whether the coalition should accept donations from liquor manufacturers and distributors to fund their substance abuse prevention services. In another African-American community, religious and philosophical differences among residents from urban and rural areas made it necessary to move a twelve-step recovery program out of a neighborhood church. The program was relocated eventually into a community center as part of its wellness program. Although some participants had already dropped out, hopefully they found other recovery programs by the time relocation occurred.

These examples highlight potential conflict areas between providers and residents and clarify the importance of providers' being aware of and effectively managing their value conflicts. Conflicts can be related to their cultural identity, knowledge about cultural education, health promotion and community-building priorities, and class and lifestyle differences.

Need to Further Refine the Framework

Afrocentric frameworks such as the one discussed in this chapter are just emerging in the literature (Schiele, 1996). African Americans' stories about their lived experiences in their communities can inform and shape the development of other frameworks and the refinement of emerging ones. The economic development arena is one in which these frameworks are being applied related to specialized areas such as entrepreneurial and welfare-to-work programs. Economic development shapes, and is influenced by, health care, housing, education, and other social policies. By implication, these emerging frameworks can provide strong guidelines for policymakers (Schiele, 1994) in funding effective economic development, community-building, and health promotion programs in African-American communities. In turn, the results of this culturally meaningful policy development and programming can highlight how these frameworks can be revised and strengthened.

Research and Evaluation Issues

A final implication is the need to use culturally relevant research and evaluation strategies for refining and disseminating the results of community-building health promotion programs in African-American communities. For instance, ethnographic, narrative, and historical research strategies may be more consistent methodologically with an Afrocentric philosophy and oral tradition (Freeman, 1999). Moreover, the framework's emphasis on full partnerships with families and other residents implies that these stakeholders' agendas and preferences should shape the planning and decision-making process for selecting research and evaluation methods. Residents should be involved, similarly, in the data gathering, analysis, and dissemination phases of community research. In this capacity-building process, providers can learn about and build upon residents' existing skills and help them to learn other skills that complement their indigenous and formal experiences.

CONCLUSION

In using health promotion community-building strategies in African-American communities, focus on individual and family change alone reinforces victim blaming and a lack of structural changes. These strategies require equal emphasis on macro interventions to address underlying institutional oppression and discrimination, and related risk factors. Community approaches are consistent with the "whole village" concept, in which, from an Afrocentric framework, comprehensive services involving residents as full partners need to be undertaken. The process is long term, as the pacing may be different in various communities where African-American residents have different values and lifestyles, and it is frequently difficult to evaluate in ways that are culturally meaningful and valuable to residents and policymakers alike. Nevertheless, it is an essential undertaking for equity purposes, and for an enhanced quality of life within African-American communities across the country.

REFERENCES

Akbar, N. (1984). Africentric social sciences for human liberation. *Journal of Black Studies, 14,* 395-414.

Asante, M.K. (1988). *Afrocentricity.* Trenton, NJ: Africa World Press.

Briar-Lawson, K., Lawson, H., Collier, C., and Joseph, A. (1997). School-linked comprehensive services: Promising beginnings, lessons learned, and future challenges. *Social Work in Education, 19*(1), 136-148.

Burwell, N.Y. (1995). Shifting the historical lens: Early economic empowerment among African Americans. *The Journal of Baccalaureate Social Work, 1*(1), 25-35.

Caplan, R.D., Vinokur, A.D., Price, R., and van Ryn, M. (1989). Job-seeking, reemployment and mental health: A randomized field experiment in coping with job loss. *Journal of Applied Psychology, 74*(4), 759-769.

Checkoway, B. (1995). Six strategies of community change. *Community Development Journal, 30*(1), 2-20.

Cox, E.O. (1991). The critical role of social action in empowerment-oriented groups. *Social Work with Groups, 14,* 77-90.

Crawley, B. and Freeman, E.M. (1993). Themes in the life views of older and younger African American males. *Journal of African American Male Studies, 1,* 15-29.

Freeman, E.M. (1999). *Culturally sensitive research strategies.* Paper presented at the Society for Social Work Research Conference, Austin, TX, February 8-10.

Freeman, E.M. and O'Dell, K. (1997). Ethnographic research methods for multicultural needs assessments: A systems change perspective. In J. Gordon (Ed.), *A systems change perspective* (pp. 55-67). New York: Mellen Press.

Gutierrez, L., Alvarez, A.R., Nemon, H., and Lewis, E.A. (1996). Multicultural community organizing: A strategy for change. *Social Work, 41*(4), 501-508.

Gutierrez, L.M. and Lewis, E.A. (1994). Community organizing with women of color: A feminist approach. *Journal of Community Practice, 1*(1), 23-44.

Hardy-Fanta, C. (1986). Social action in Hispanic groups. *Social Work, 31*(2), 119-123.

Harris, N. (1992). A philosophical basis for an Afrocentric orientation. *Western Journal of Black Studies, 16*(2), 154-159.

Kirst, M. (1996). School-linked services. Pitfalls and potentials. *Spectrum 1,* 15-24.

Melaville, A.I. and Blank, M.J. (1993). *Together we can: A guide for crafting a profamily system of education and human services.* Report prepared for the U.S. Department of Education, Office of Educational Research and Improvement, and U.S. Department of Health and Human Services, Office of the Assistant Secretary of Planning and Evaluation. Washington, DC: U.S. Government Printing Office.

Nobles, W.W. (1980). African philosophy: Foundations for black psychology. In R. Jones (Ed.), *Black psychology* (Third edition) (pp. 23-35). New York: Harper & Row.

Oliver, W. (1989). Black males and social problems: Prevention through Africentric socialization. *Journal of Black Studies, 20*(1), 15-39.

Poole, D. (1995). Beyond the rhetoric: Shared responsibility versus the Contract with America. (Editorial). *Health and Social Work, 20,* 83-86.

Raheim, S. and Bolden, J. (1995). Economic empowerment of low-income women through self-employment programs. *Affilia, 10,* 138-154.

Read, M. (1992). Drug treatment with dually diagnosed clients. In E.M. Freeman (Ed.), *Substance abuse treatment: A family systems perspective* (pp. 56-78). Newbury Park, CA: Sage.

Saleebey, D. (1996). *The strengths perspective in social work practice* (Second edition). White Plains, NY: Longman.

Schiele, J.H. (1990). Organizational theory from an Afrocentric perspective. *Journal of Black Studies, 21*(2), 145-161.

Schiele, J.H. (1994). Afrocentricity as an alternative world view for equality. *Journal of Progressive Human Services, 5*(1), 5-25.

Schiele, J.H. (1996). Afrocentricity: An emerging paradigm in social work practice. *Social Work, 41*(2), 284-294.

Solomon, B. (1987). *Empowerment: Social work in oppressed communities.* New York: Columbia University Press.

Weick, A. (1985). Overturning the medical model. *Social Work, 30*(2), 310-315.

Weil, M. (1996). Community building: Building community practice. *Social Work, 41*(3), 481-500.

Weil, M. and Gamble, D. (1995). Community practice models. In R.L. Edwards (Ed.), *Encyclopedia of social work* (Nineteenth edition) (pp. 577-593). Washington, DC: NASW.

PART IV:
EPILOGUE

Chapter 14

A View Toward the Future: Implications for Empowerment Practice, Research, and Policy Development in the Black Community

Edith M. Freeman
Sadye L. Logan

In some ways, many of the chapters in this book capture the essence of the Nigerian proverb that reflects the dilemma African-American communities are confronted with today: "He who is being carried does not realize how far the village is." Many of the social supports and policies that were designed to replace the cultural institutions that had been destroyed during slavery have, in fact, robbed African Americans of their self-determination. What was initially a temporary solution has become the problem, with chronic, systemic, and debilitating effects. Those effects have had the greatest impact in areas that are essential for any community's survival, in health, education, economics, and politics.

One result has been the loss of the village concept and a viable spirituality, whereby some residents no longer have a sense of social, ethical, and cultural responsibility for the group. The strong spiritual support and traditional cultural interdependence among community members has been replaced, in some instances, with dependence on government institutions, as reflected in the aforementioned proverb. Consequently, black communities are currently at a crossroad, where survival alone, although a triumph in the past, is not sufficient in today's climate. Black communities are at a point at which they can go forward or slide backward, but where standing still is not an option. Major changes have occurred and will continue to occur because of many internal and external forces. The journey ahead is similar to the twin Chinese symbols for crisis: it will be filled with both opportunities and risks for black communities.

POTENTIAL OPPORTUNITIES AND RISKS FOR BLACK COMMUNITIES

Opportunities and Resources

Opportunities can include time for regrouping, for sorting through the critical issues that are confronting black communities today and alternatives that are available for addressing those issues. Subgroups within these communities have different, sometimes conflicting, values and ideas about priority issues and viable alternatives. Those differences may be based on a combination of factors, such as age, socioeconomic status, lifestyle, gender, geographic region, political ideology, the number of family generations born in this country, and the country from which a family emigrated. For these reasons, establishing a common vision and agenda within each black community will be challenging, but the process can lead to collective healing and growth.

Reassessments of black communities' strengths, resiliency, and other assets across within-group differences is another important opportunity. Since the combination of subgroups within each of these communities is unique, creativity will be required to build on that uniqueness. Reestablishing the village concept as part of this creative process can help in community building by strengthening vital components of communities' infrastructure, such as leadership, economic, and political development. The journey toward strengthening and, in some communities, toward building the infrastructure, can only occur if those communities reestablish a cultural and social responsibility for the group as a whole.

Potential Risks

In contrast to the previous opportunities, the current crossroad for black communities involves a number of potential risks. Those risks can diminish the opportunities and the incredible resilience that are present within black communities. One risk is that those communities might be swayed by and begin to believe media sooth-sayers who are predicting the swift demise of black communities. Those predictions ignore the history of black communities in taking care of their own and in coping with, and successfully advocating against, systemic barriers such as institutional racism.

Another risk is that black communities will forget the lessons learned from the civil rights era and the institution of slavery. Those lessons include the importance of maintaining a balance between "going it alone" and building coalitions with other ethnic and socio-economic groups. Some issues confronting black communities are appropriate for those communities to handle alone, such as the mentoring of black boys, whereas other issues require mobilization with other groups, such as advocating against hate groups and hate crimes.

The lack of accessible health care resources is a risk that can affect all life domains in impoverished and black communities, if it is not addressed effectively, now and in the future. As discussed throughout this book, substance abuse, community violence, and chronic illnesses such as diabetes, hypertension, and heart disease are examples of conditions that pose increasingly high risks for black communities. In the face of these escalating health conditions, recent social policy reforms and the failure of the U.S. Congress to pass a national health care bill for the poor have decreased health care resources for black communities. These risks and the related opportunities should be considered as future empowerment practice, research, and policy development occur in black communities.

IMPLICATIONS FOR FUTURE EMPOWERMENT PRACTICE

Future practice in black communities should encompass formal service programs and mutual help supports. A common consideration across both types of service provision is the need to plan for within-group differences that can affect how problems and strengths are defined, consumers' roles in the helping process are envisioned, the type and amount of change that is consistent with consumers' values, and who is expected to provide the services.

Formal Empowerment Programs/Practice

Culturally meaningful interventions for black communities should be philosophically compatible with the worldviews, beliefs, and values of the residents. Those interventions should focus on goals related to capacity building and systems changes, to address risk conditions identified in the previous section. Including mezzo and macro interventions can help service providers avoid labeling community residents as the cause of community and large systems problems. The residents in those communities should be viewed as experts on their life situations, communities, and experiences. Based on that assumption, the residents should be involved actively in assessing their communities' strengths and needs, and in planning, implementing, and evaluating empowerment programs that develop from those assessments. The within-group diversity in those communities should be viewed as a strength by service planners and providers.

This partnership process can encourage black communities to participate in deciding on the type of cultural programs that are needed to fit the unique combination of subgroups within communities. Some in black communities may want mainstream programs that address some aspects of cultural differences, while including generic components for people of all ethnic groups. Other communities may want more culturally relevant empowerment programs. In such programs, interventions are provided for addressing systemic economic and political barriers to health and for helping residents apply Afrocentric values, philosophy, and traditions to their daily lives in the community.

Community Mutual Help Supports

Empowerment practice should include practitioners facilitating black communities in identifying the need for and developing mutual help resources. Areas typically addressed by such supports in black communities in the past include leadership development, mentoring of the young, economic development, and political activism and systems changes. These resources can help black communities to reestablish the village concept in the future, and to apply African principles that are consistent with the concept of collectivism or mutual responsibility. Such resources can also reinforce the concept of the residents as experts and their communities as resilient.

IMPLICATIONS FOR FUTURE RESEARCH

Researchers in black communities will need to develop principles for conducting studies that are consistent with the values of these communities, such as Montgomery-Rice and Richard-Davis have reported in this book (see Chapter 6), recognizing that there will be within-group differences. Those principles should focus on the researchers' philosophy about appropriate methods and the role of community residents, the cultural relevance of the interventions under study, and the meaning of the research data to community residents.

The Researchers' Philosophy/Role of Residents

The use of research paradigms and methods that emphasize a participatory, consumer-driven, and culturally oriented process is of critical importance (Gilgun, 1994). Hence, researchers in black communities should be aware of the effects of their social perspectives or philosophies on the research process and outcomes. A researcher's pathology or deficit paradigm or his or her ethnocentrism is likely to result in findings that emphasize community pathology, without consideration of systemic barriers or the residents' strengths. Researchers should involve such communities in identifying research questions that are culturally meaningful to them and methods that are consistent with their values and ways of viewing the world. In this way, residents can use their expertise to identify their communities' strengths and resources, how those assets can be utilized during the research, and viable roles for residents in the research process.

Study of Interventions' Cultural Relevance

Future research in black communities should also explore, modify interventions as needed, and disseminate information about the cultural relevance of interventions that are under study. This principle implies that research questions related to those communities should always include a focus on the participants' views about the meaningfulness of the services provided (Burman and Allen-Meares, 1991; Freeman, 1991). It also implies that the researcher should listen actively for information from the participants about their cultural values, worldviews, traditions, and rituals as the context for understanding their conclusions about the cultural relevance of the services.

Cultural Meanings in Terms of Findings

Research in black communities should involve mechanisms for exploring the meaning of the data to residents. As noted previously, including residents in assessing their needs and strengths is merely a foundation for structuring research so that it is more likely to yield meaningful results for the stakeholders. In later phases of the research, focus groups, interviews, or written summaries of preliminary findings can be used to do member checking with the residents (Lincoln, 1995). This process raises questions with residents about the accuracy of the data and how they should be interpreted from a cultural perspective and addresses differences that may develop as residents struggle with those questions. Moreover, questions should be raised during the process about how the data can be used, which parts of the findings should be disseminated, in what format, and to whom.

POLICY IMPLICATIONS

Dissemination can be a tool for helping black communities to influence policy development that supports their efforts toward self-determination in the future. Information to be disseminated can come from the formal research discussed in the previous section or from informal data from residents' lived experiences. Informal data about communities' strengths and resilience can supplement formal research data that may be biased toward emphasizing problems out of their context. Dissemination to policymakers on the long- and short-term health needs and effective interventions is critical for helping to shape the development of strengths-focused social policies. According to Chapin (1995), this strategy leads to policies that do not shift from labeling problems to labeling people as the problem.

Policies that affect black communities must also consider the role of the environment in creating or reinforcing the risks that are confronting those communities today. Such policies should include opportunities and resources for helping black communities to strengthen their infrastructure in terms of leadership, economic, and political development. Policies that do not facilitate the black community's economic development only provide short-term token opportunities for improved functioning. Those policies provide, for example, low-income, non-career-ladder work training in black communities, without changing the economic system itself or without leading to communities' economic well-being and health in the long term.

CONCLUSION

A major theme in this book is one that is rooted in systems theory and its concepts. The book emphasizes, for example, that the health of black families and communities is closely related to how they function in their other life domains, in mental health, economic, and political domains. The book also clarifies the role of systems in creating and reinforcing environmental barriers to black families' and communities' health and well-being, or, in some circumstances, in supporting or hindering their strengths.

The current combination of risks and opportunities can, indeed, become a turning point for African-American families and communities. This turning point can include the realignment of systemic forces to help these communities recognize and act upon their potential for self-determination and cultural synergy.

REFERENCES

Burman, S. and Allen-Meares, P. (1991). Criteria for selecting practice theories: Working with alcoholic women. *Families in Society, 72*(3), 387-393.

Chapin, R.K. (1995). Social policy development: The strengths perspective. *Social Work, 40*(3), 483-495.

Freeman, E.M. (1991). Social competence as a framework for addressing ethnicity and teenage alcohol problems. In A.R. Stiffman and L.E. Davis (Eds.), *Ethnic issues in adolescent mental health* (pp. 247-266). Newbury Park, CA: Sage.

Gilgun, J.F. (1994). A case for case studies in social work research. *Social Work, 39*(2), 371-380.

Lincoln, Y.S. (1995). Emerging criteria for quality in qualitative and interpretive research. *Qualitative Inquiry, 3*(2), 275-289.

Index

Page numbers followed by the letter "f" indicate figures; those followed by the letter "t" indicate tables.

Order Your Own Copy of
This Important Book for Your Personal Library!

HEALTH CARE IN THE BLACK COMMUNITY
Empowerment, Knowledge, Skills, and Collectivism

_____ in hardbound at $69.95 (ISBN: 0-7890-0456-9)

_____ in softbound at $34.95 (ISBN: 0-7890-0457-7)

COST OF BOOKS_____

OUTSIDE USA/CANADA/
MEXICO: ADD 20%_____

POSTAGE & HANDLING_____
(US: $4.00 for first book & $1.50
for each additional book
Outside US: $5.00 for first book
& $2.00 for each additional book)

SUBTOTAL_____

IN CANADA: ADD 7% GST_____

STATE TAX_____
(NY, OH & MN residents, please
add appropriate local sales tax)

FINAL TOTAL_____
(If paying in Canadian funds,
convert using the current
exchange rate. UNESCO
coupons welcome.)

☐ **BILL ME LATER:** ($5 service charge will be added)
(Bill-me option is good on US/Canada/Mexico orders only;
not good to jobbers, wholesalers, or subscription agencies.)

☐ Check here if billing address is different from
shipping address and attach purchase order and
billing address information.

Signature_____

☐ **PAYMENT ENCLOSED: $**_____

☐ **PLEASE CHARGE TO MY CREDIT CARD.**

☐ Visa   ☐ MasterCard   ☐ AmEx   ☐ Discover
☐ Diner's Club   ☐ Eurocard   ☐ JCB

Account # _____

Exp. Date _____

Signature _____

Prices in US dollars and subject to change without notice.

NAME _____
INSTITUTION _____
ADDRESS _____
CITY _____
STATE/ZIP _____
COUNTRY _____ COUNTY (NY residents only) _____
TEL _____ FAX _____
E-MAIL_____
May we use your e-mail address for confirmations and other types of information? ☐ Yes   ☐ No
We appreciate receiving your e-mail address and fax number. Haworth would like to e-mail or fax special
discount offers to you, as a preferred customer. **We will never share, rent, or exchange your e-mail
address or fax number.** We regard such actions as an invasion of your privacy.

Order From Your Local Bookstore or Directly From
The Haworth Press, Inc.
10 Alice Street, Binghamton, New York 13904-1580 • USA
TELEPHONE: 1-800-HAWORTH (1-800-429-6784) / Outside US/Canada: (607) 722-5857
FAX: 1-800-895-0582 / Outside US/Canada: (607) 772-6362
E-mail: getinfo@haworthpressinc.com
PLEASE PHOTOCOPY THIS FORM FOR YOUR PERSONAL USE.
www.HaworthPress.com

BOF00

362.1   Health care in the
Hea   Black community.

DATE			

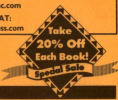